PRAISE FOR THE ORIGINAL EDITION
OF *GOOD CARBS, BAD CARBS*

"This book is written for all those sensible folks who harbor doubts about the wisdom of low-carb diets. Here are the facts written into a simple, no-nonsense guide which shows you how your brain and your body will benefit from good carbs."

—Professor Jennie Brand-Miller,
coauthor of *The New Glucose Revolution*

"A diet that doesn't demonize carbohydrates? Love it!... One of the few books in our rankings to get the GI science right.... Bottom line: Good book; good-bye elastic waistband.... A–"

—*Self*

Johanna Burani, M.S., R.D., C.D.E.

Good Carbs,

LOSE WEIGHT AND ENJOY OPTIMUM
HEALTH AND VITALITY BY EATING
THE *RIGHT* CARBS

Bad Carbs

SECOND EDITION—REVISED & UPDATED

MARLOWE & COMPANY
NEW YORK

*To Sergio, for teaching me about
selflessness and patience;*

*To Matteo, for teaching me about
trust and conviction;*

*To Paul, for teaching me about
generosity and sincerity;*

*To Dad, for teaching me
about integrity and love;*

*And to Mom, my first and best teacher.
You all are the wind beneath my wings.*

Thank you.

> *Let thy food be thy medicine.*

—Hippocrates

CONTENTS

Contents

PART 3
Recipes

PREFACE

This book replaces a visit to my office. For nearly two decades, I have provided nutrition counseling, hand-holding, and even an occasional tissue to the most wonderful people in the world, my patients.

Some people come to me for weight loss, or diabetes management, or for elevated cholesterol or blood pressure; some have gastrointestinal problems or are just poor or fussy eaters. Many arrive fearful, confused, anxious, angry, depressed; others haven't a clue *why* they've come, in fact they really don't want to see me at all, but they've come at the insistence of their spouse or doctor.

What usually winds up happening after our first visit is, for me, the most gratifying part of my work day: the patient leaves with a clear, practical "game plan" of how to eat better, and, thus, how to begin to address the fears, confusion, anxiety, anger and depression stemming from their health concerns. We talk about how to do something constructive and beneficial for both the body and the mind. The focus is placed on something as simple and familiar as mindfully eating a healthful meal. In one short visit, the "good diet" has been demystified and brought right onto that person's next dinner plate!

So, in this book I've written down (and expanded upon) what I tell my patients face-to-face. You'll notice that I've written in a conversational style, as if you were, in fact, in my office with me; as if you were, in fact, my patient.

Good Carbs, Bad Carbs was written in September 2001. As in the world at large, so too in the field of nutrition, much has changed since then. This revised edition updates health statistics (which, sadly, have not improved in the interim), discusses new health initiatives, like the 10,000-Steps Program (see page 90), provides expanded lists of reference and interactive Web sites, and discusses topics or concerns pertinent to our present nutrition dialogue, like upcoming changes to the Dietary Guidelines for Americans, the Food Guide Pyramid, and, of course, the high-protein craze. I've also included more recipes at the unremitting insistence of my patients.

This book provides a basic overview of carbohydrates: how they work, what they do in and for the body, why they hold such a privileged position in the balanced diet, and how they contribute to good health. A major theme, namely *"carbohydrates are the body's fuel of choice,"* runs throughout this book and I'm hoping it will become a welcomed new mantra for you!

Don't worry, though, you're not holding a textbook nor is *Good Carbs, Bad Carbs* a definitive book on carbohydrates. But if you've heard about carbs before and you'd like to learn more about how they can benefit you, then this book is for you!

I tell my patients that there are no bad foods, just bad diets. So, in spite of the title, *Good Carbs, Bad Carbs*, there are no really bad carbs. But there is no argument about some foods giving your body quality calories while others just provide empty ones. The same holds for carbohydrate foods. Carbohydrates are important because the body selectively chooses them as its preferred fuel source. And eating the *right*, or let's say *better or "smarter"* carbs, which you will quickly learn are the more slowly digested ones, can help you control blood-glucose levels (believe it or not, a concern for everyone, not just people with diabetes), give you enough energy to sustain your mental alertness and physical activitiy throughout the day, help you achieve a healthy weight and even boost your heart's health. This book is about those carbs. And I've written it just for you!

And to help you make the best carb choices when you are out food shopping, I've included a tear-out food guide. It's the next best thing to having me there to help you choose wisely for your health. I hope you'll consult this card whenever you enter a food store and as you're making decisions about what food to eat.

A Book in Two Parts

As you scan the contents, you'll see that the book is divided into two parts. In part 1 I describe what carbs are: how they work and how your well-being and good health are affected by the amount, and type, of carbohydrates you eat.

Part 2 describes how eating slowly digested carbs can impact on weight loss, diabetes, and heart health. I'm not suggesting that eating carbohydrates *alone* can prevent diseases; no food by itself can do that. My goal is to point out that eating the *right kind* of carbs can positively influence many diseases. In addition, part 2 also gives you the heads-up on carb intake as it relates to children and sports nutrition.

Now, after reading that part 2 covers how carbs influence certain diseases, you might be tempted to start reading the book there. But please don't. Start with part 1, because the information there lays the foundation for what you'll read later on. If you start at the beginning, you'll better understand the terms I use throughout this book and exactly how certain carbs work to positively affect your health.

Why You Need This Book

If you think that you're already pretty healthy—you don't have diabetes or heart disease or need to lose weight—you may wonder what this book has to offer you. Well, do a quick mental survey. Do you feel an energy dip mid-afternoon? Do you ever need to raid the fridge between meals because you feel hungry? Do you think that you could be eating better? If you answered "yes" to any of these questions, then this book may help you. And if you already suffer from overweight, diabetes, or heart disease, I'll show you how you can better manage your condition, reduce your risk of further complications, and feel much better too!

To your good health.

Johanna Burani, M.S., R.D., C.D.E.

PART 1

Carbohydrates: Your Body's Fuel of Choice

1

A BALANCED DIET DEFINED

Even though some food advertisements may claim otherwise, no one food will protect you from poor health. And as unhealthful as some foods may be, no one food will kill you. In fact, there really are no bad foods—just bad diets. There are also good diets. How can you recognize the difference? And what is a diet anyway?

Diets vs. Diet

Who isn't tired of hearing and thinking about how to lose weight? We are diet-hounded by every possible media source, by people around us, maybe even by our doctors, and very likely, if we are among the majority of Americans who currently admit to the need to lose weight, by our own inner voices. Maybe you have tried one (or more) of the low-carb, or low-fat, or low-calorie routes, just like millions of other Americans who are presently battling their bulge.

Who isn't also tired of hearing and thinking about the doom and gloom statistics of weight loss failures? Eighty-five to ninety-five percent of all dieters are reportedly unsuccessful in maintaining their weight loss, although it must be stated that this is a conjecture and not based on hard clinically proven facts. Truth be told, the National Weight Control Registry (see page 67) offers us much better odds at successful weight-loss maintenance. Nonetheless, many dieters never reach their weight-loss goals. Who/what failed: the dieter or the diet?

As a nutrition counselor, the word "diet" is used many times throughout my workday. I learned a long time ago that my definition of the word is different from that of my patients. Most people equate a diet primarily with losing weight; they see it as something they go "on" and, when they go "off" it, they are "cheating" or are "bad." So, they go "on" 1,000-calorie diets, low-carb diets, no-fat diets, or whatever else is the latest weight-loss trend. My nutrition textbooks taught me that a diet is a way of eating, one's normal choice of foods, a lifestyle, a behavior that is effortlessly perpetuated. And so, I encourage a healthful, balanced **diet** that excludes no one food or food group but stresses wholesome foods and reasonable portions as well as palatability and enjoyment. How else to promote nutritious eating habits, that is to say, **a healthful diet?**

There is nothing wrong with the dieters I have met in my practice. There is usually a lot wrong with their dietary attempts to lose weight. The failure is in the **diet** not the **dieter.**

What Does "Diet" Mean?

The tenth edition of *Merriam Webster's Collegiate Dictionary* defines the noun *diet* as "food and drink regularly provided or consumed."

(By the way, some dictionaries also provide a second definition of *diet*: "to restrict oneself to special food, esp. in order to control one's weight; to feed esp. on special food as treatment or punishment." While dieting—by this definition anyway—can certainly feel like punishment, it isn't a nutritionist's working definition!)

This book is a book about healthy eating for optimal health. So in dietitians' lingo, that makes it a diet book! It explains how, with the right food choices, your normal, everyday diet can help you achieve and maintain good health. It provides you with a clear explanation of why carbohydrates are the single most influential nutrient in your diet—a diet that affects your day-to-day living, as well as your general health.

The 40-Plus Diet
(aka A Balanced Diet)

Let's start with the idea of a *balanced diet*. A balanced diet supports your good health by supplying you with the 40-plus nutrients that your body needs every day. It consists of a wide variety of nutrient-dense, healthful foods. (Nutrient-dense foods, by the way, are those foods that offer a lot of the good things your body needs—such as calcium, fiber, and protein, for example—for the calories it receives.) A balanced diet contains carbohydrates, protein, fat, vitamins, minerals, and water. We can think of each of these nutrients functioning as a team player, with the carbohydrate foods in the diet playing the role of team captain.

Keeping all of these nutrients in mind when you're selecting foods from a restaurant menu or a supermarket shelf may seem like a tall order. It becomes easier, even *habitual*, though, when you focus on your health, at least most of the time. To assist you, the U.S. departments of Agriculture (USDA) and Health and Human Services (HHS) have published *Dietary Guidelines for Americans* to help all Americans focus on making healthful dietary and lifestyle choices. Updated every five years to reflect the most current information, the fifth edition of these guidelines was published in 2000. As this book goes to press, the latest revisions of the sixth edition are in their final stage of discussion.

Dietary Guidelines for Americans

Need help making healthful lifestyle choices? Here is the 2005 edition of the *proposed* guidelines:

➤ Consume a variety of foods within and among the basic food groups while staying within energy needs.
➤ Control calorie intake to manage body weight.
➤ Be physically active every day.
➤ Increase daily intake of fruits and vegetables, whole grains, and nonfat or low-fat milk and milk products.

> Choose fats wisely for good health.
> Choose carbohydrates wisely for good health.
> Choose and prepare foods with little salt.
> If you drink alcoholic beverages, do so in moderation.
> Keep food safe to eat.

✔ **USDA Fact**: The average American can get a full day's worth of adequate vegetables and fruits by spending just 64 cents.

These recommendations certainly provide us with a blueprint for healthful living that, based on current medical knowledge and research information, support good, even optimal health. The third recommendation, "Let the Pyramid guide your food choices," calls our attention to the Food Guide Pyramid, another informational tool presented by the USDA and HHS to help all of us put healthful eating into practice.

Diagram of the Food Guide Pyramid

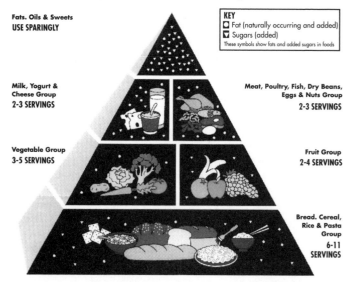

Fats. Oils & Sweets
USE SPARINGLY

KEY
☐ Fat (naturally occurring and added)
☑ Sugars (added)
These symbols show fats and added sugars in foods

Milk, Yogurt &
Cheese Group
2-3 SERVINGS

Meat, Poultry, Fish, Dry Beans,
Eggs & Nuts Group
2-3 SERVINGS

Vegetable Group
3-5 SERVINGS

Fruit Group
2-4 SERVINGS

Bread. Cereal,
Rice & Pasta
Group
6-11
SERVINGS

Source: United States Department of Agriculture and United States Department of Health and Human Services

Components of a Healthful Diet

Nutrient	Purpose	Food sources
TEAM CAPTAIN Carbohydrates	Serve as your body's primary energy source	Cereals, pasta, rice, barley, potatoes, corn, legumes, fruits, vegetables, milk, and milk products
THE TEAM PLAYERS Fats	Serve as the stored-energy form that your body draws from when there aren't enough available carbs	Oils, butter, margarine, cream, regular cream cheese, ice cream, salad dressings and mayonnaise, and the naturally occurring fat in red meat, fish, poultry, egg yolks, cheese, milk, milk products, seeds, and nuts
Proteins	Provide building blocks for organs, tissues, skin, bones, enzymes, and hormones	Red meat, fish, poultry, egg whites, cheese, tofu, milk and milk products, legumes, and nuts
Vitamins	Help your body develop and function normally; may guard against disease	Grains, fruits, vegetables, dairy products, all meats, fish and poultry, oils, nuts, and seeds
Minerals	Help your body develop and function normally; may guard against disease	Grains, fruits, vegetables, dairy products, all meats, fish and poultry, oils, nuts, and seeds
Water	Needed for all metabolic activities; helps transport glucose and other vital nutrients to cells; helps eliminate cellular waste products; helps you maintain a constant body temperature	Liquids such as water, juice, milk, soda, non-caffeinated beverages; to a lesser extent, water is in virtually all foods

You can see how the Food Pyramid goes hand in hand with the food recommendations of the *Dietary Guidelines*. Both of these tools stress the importance of eating balanced meals that contain a variety of nutrient-dense foods and moderate portion sizes. Both tools are designed to help you make eating a healthful *diet* a healthful *habit*.

The Food Guide Pyramid clearly stresses the importance of selecting foods from all the food groups. And while you need all groups for the best possible health, the Pyramid shows that the foundation of a healthful diet should come from grains (especially whole-grain breads and cereals, rice, and pasta, as you'll see emphasized throughout this book). The Pyramid also shows that you should be eating several servings of fruits and vegetables and dairy every day; in fact, some nutritionists believe that as much as 75 percent of your daily food servings should come from these four high-carbohydrate food groups. The fact is, eating whole grains, fruits, vegetables, and low-fat dairy foods does seem to be the easiest way to get the carbohydrates, as well as the protein, vitamins, minerals, fiber, and water you need without overdoing the amount of fat. Because you need fats from your diet, it's best to choose the heart-healthful kinds (mono- and polyunsaturated) as often as possible from foods such as vegetable oils, fish, nuts, and seeds. For more on dietary fats and heart health, see chapter 7.

There is some discussion currently going on in the health and nutrition arenas about future restructuring of the Food Guide Pyramid. Some experts believe that a strong statement should be made to include exercise and weight control as a primary focus of a healthful diet. They also suggest a more prominent positioning of whole grains, plant oils, fruits and vegetables, nuts, and legumes than is seen on the current Food Pyramid. By default, dairy foods, red meat, refined grains, butter, and sweets would all be given a less significant status in contributing to a balanced diet. The Food Guide Pyramid initiative has served us well thus far in establishing carbohydrate-based foods as the foundation of the most healthful, balanced diet. The thrust toward more whole grains, more fruits and vegetables, and legumes, I believe, is an appropriate fine-tuning next step. This book gives you all the reasons why.

By the way, if you are interested in learning more about the science behind the new restructuring suggestions for the Food Guide Pyramid, take a look at Dr. Walter Willett's book, published in 2001, *Eat, Drink and Be Healthy.*

Your Diet: The Role Carbs Play

So all of this interest in grains, fruits, vegetables, and dairy in your diet puts these high-carbohydrate foods front and center on the good-nutrition stage. But how and why did these carbs get all this attention in the first place? If most of your food selections should come from these food groups, it's important to understand what your body gets from them.

First of all, let me repeat: You need protein, fat, vitamins, minerals, and water as well as carbohydrates to be healthy, and many foods offer an abundance of these vital nutrients. All of these nutrients play an important role in a well-balanced diet. So why are carbs so critical? *Because they are your body's fuel of choice.*

Your body prefers to get its energy from the carbohydrates you eat rather than from either proteins or fats. Without going into the chemical explanation of why carbs get this special treatment (that comes later), for now, let's just say that your body recognizes that carbohydrates contain the greatest potential for providing immediate energy. Somehow, your body knows that it's going to wind up with more glucose flowing in the bloodstream after you eat carbs than it will after you eat either proteins or fats. And it wants to get as much energy as it can with the least amount of work.

So what do you get when you eat high-carbohydrate foods? You get most of the energy you need for all your daily activities.

Carb Food Sources

High-carbohydrate foods include cereals, grains, legumes (such as lentils and kidney beans), fruits, vegetables, and milk products. Not coincidentally, most of these foods make up the bottom layers of the Food Guide Pyramid.

Your Diet: The Role Fat Plays

When it comes to getting quick energy from food, your body ignores dietary fats, although they do make an important contribution by providing you with the form of energy you can easily store to use later. Here's how fat storage works: Of all the nutrients you eat, fats contain the most calories. And because of the chemical structure of these calories, your body chooses them as its favorite nutrient for body-fat storage. In fact, your body has been programmed, throughout evolution, to store *dietary* fats as *body* fat, for use in a possible future famine. Because most of us don't usually go hungry for more than a few hours at a time (or at all), we don't usually have a chance to dip into this stored fat for energy. Instead, you already know where it all goes: on your thighs, around your middle, and on your butt!

So, from fats, your body gets its best energy reserves. In fact, your body just loves to store fat and has an almost unlimited capacity to do so. The more fat stores it has, the happier it is. Not great news, is it? But this storage capacity explains why it's such a good idea to cut back on fats if you're trying to lose weight.

Fat Food Sources

Sources of dietary fats include red meat, fish, poultry, egg yolks, cheese (except nonfat), milk and milk products (except nonfat), butter, margarine, and oils, cream, ice cream, regular cream cheese and salad dressings, mayonnaise (except nonfat), seeds, and nuts.

Your Diet: The Role Protein Plays

Dietary proteins have a privileged status in your body: Protein foods provide the only building blocks your body uses to restore and repair itself. If your body were forced to use protein for energy because there weren't enough available carbs—its preferred fuel—it could; and it does, in extreme cases, such as during prolonged starvation. But breaking down protein for energy is a more complicated process and not one that your body easily performs.

So, from protein foods, your body gets the building units to make and maintain your organs, muscles, skin, tissues, and your entire lean body mass. Protein is vital for a healthy body, but watch out: Eat too many protein calories and your body won't make stronger or bigger muscles out of them—it will make body fat.

Protein Food Sources

The main protein sources include red meat, fish, poultry, egg whites, cheese, tofu, milk and milk products, as well as legumes and nuts.

So, at the end of the day, just what do you get from eating a well-balanced diet?

- Balanced proportions of carbohydrate (55 to 60 percent), protein (10 to 15 percent) and fat (less than 30 percent)
- Enough calories to meet your energy needs for the day
- At least the minimum amounts of most, if not all, of the 40-plus nutrients you need for good health

---

THE BOTTOM LINE

➤ A diet is how we normally eat.

➤ A balanced diet supports good health by supplying you with the 40-plus nutrients that you need every day.

➤ Carbohydrates are your body's fuel of choice.

➤ Carbs give you the imediate energy you need for all of your daily activities.

➤ Fats are used by the body to store energy.

➤ Proteins are used by the body to restore and repair itself.

2

How Carbs Work

Carbs, because they serve such an important function in your body, require some explanation. And though I've done my best to simplify some very technical information, I know that for some people, this chapter won't exactly be a page-turner. But the concepts are relatively easy to understand, so hang in there. Because, once you have a basic understanding of the facts in this chapter, you'll be able to better appreciate why carbs are the most important nutrient for everyday life. Ready? Let's go!

All of your body's functions, from breathing to moving to thinking, come from the energy that food molecules produce within your cells. That's why food has a direct bearing on how well your body feels and works. But what are these molecules? What do they look like? What do they do?

Molecules Made Simple

Molecules are just tiny units from which everything around us is made—dogs and cats, sunflowers and bees, and the foods we eat. Your body is also composed of trillions of molecules. What makes up a carbohydrate molecule? When you think of how many thousands, tens of thousands, of different carbohydrate-containing foods there are (like potatoes, chocolate chip cookies, apples, milk shakes, and pizza) it's almost shocking to learn that they all contain just three basic units, called atoms: carbon (C), oxygen (O), and hydrogen (H). In fact, that's how carbs get their name:

carbo = carbon (C)
hydrate = with water (H_2O)

These atoms join together (or bond) to form carbohydrate molecules. The different sizes and shapes of these carbohydrate molecules give special characteristics to the foods they're in. For example, carbohydrates in bread have a different chemical structure and size than carbohydrates in peaches—and that's why bread and peaches look and taste different to us. But because these molecules are made of carbon, oxygen, and hydrogen, they are all carbohydrates.

The Simple Carbohydrates

Simple carbohydrates are all sugars and fall into two categories: (1) one-molecule, or single sugars, or (2) two-molecule, or double sugars. The scientific names for these sugars are monosaccharides and disaccharides respectively. The most important monosaccharides are *glucose, fructose,* and *galactose.* The most important disaccharides are *maltose, sucrose,* and *lactose.* Your body breaks these double sugars down into at least one molecule of glucose and another single sugar.

In fact, this book is all about glucose: where it comes from in your diet and how you get it from the food you eat, what your body does with it, and why it prefers to use carbohydrates to get it.

The Monosaccharides: Glucose

Glucose, your body's "gasoline," is the most important of all the sugars in your system. It's the form of sugar that flows through your blood to provide energy to your cells; it also serves as the structural unit of glycogen, one of your body's stored energy forms.

As a sugar, glucose tastes mildly sweet and occurs naturally in foods such as fruit and honey. In your body, it's hard to exaggerate glucose's importance: No other substance is more essential. Glucose is the form of energy that travels into your cells, allowing them to do their individual jobs. Every activity that every body cell performs occurs because of glucose. No glucose, no life. Now, *that's* how important it is!

What Do these Things Mean?

Troubled by some of the technical terms you see? Here is how those words break down into simple meanings:

mono = one

di = two

poly = many

saccharide = sugar

ose = sugar in

The Monosaccharides: Fructose

Fructose, also known as fruit sugar, is naturally found in all fruits, honey, and tree saps. It's the sweetest-tasting of all the naturally occurring sugars; you'll find it as an ingredient in some jellies, ice cream, cookies, yogurt, and sweets. With a little help from your liver, fructose can convert into the all-important energizer, glucose, or it can be stored as the starch glycogen. And, if your glycogen stores are all filled up, you can also store fructose as fat.

What Is High-Fructose Corn Syrup?

This popular food ingredient is an intensely sweet sugar that food companies use to manufacture certain sweetened beverages, baked and frozen desserts, and some preserved foods, such as relishes and maraschino cherries. (To learn more about how high-fructose corn syrup may be linked to weight gain and type 2 diabetes, see pages 114–117)

The Monosaccharides: Galactose

This sugar helps to form the disaccharide lactose, which is important because it is the sugar naturally occurring in milk, an essential part of a balanced diet. Galactose is also a component of several bulking agents and stabilizers, such as carrageenan and guar gum, which are commonly used in many commercially prepared dessert and confectionery products.

Single sugars (Monosaccharides)

	Purpose	Found in
Glucose	Your body's number-one source of immediate energy; any excess will be stored as glycogen	Fruit, honey, sugar
Fructose	Converted to glucose in the liver, for energy use as needed	Fruit, honey, tree sap, sugar
Galactose	Converted to glucose in the liver, for energy use as needed	Milk and milk products, bulking agents used in chewing gum and ice cream

The Disaccharides: Maltose

Maltose, also called malt sugar, isn't used very often as a food ingredient. But here are two important things to know about maltose: First, it's a disaccharide made of two glucose molecules. More simply put, your body takes one molecule of maltose and makes two glucose molecules out of it. Second, anytime you digest starch, your body breaks down the starch into maltose, which then breaks down into glucose. So on any given day, if you're eating a balanced diet as prescribed by the Food Guide Pyramid, you're taking in quite a few starch molecules. Your body easily digests 100 percent of these molecules into the sugar it's searching for—glucose.

White Bread's Tale

Have you ever let a piece of sliced white bread linger in your mouth long enough for the enzymes there to start digestion? If you did, you'd soon realize that the bread was starting to taste sweet, not starchy. What makes it sweet? The bread starch begins to break down into smaller and smaller molecules until the sugar (maltose) forms, which then breaks down further into two glucose molecules. That's where the sweetness comes from. Try it sometime!

The Disaccharides: Sucrose

Sucrose is another name for table sugar. It is also called beet sugar or cane sugar. It is found naturally in some plant juices or saps, such as pure maple syrup. It's the sugar you're most familiar with: you put it in your tea or coffee, or sprinkled on your breakfast cereal; you bake and cook with it and you are likely to ingest it in some of the commercially prepared foods you may consume throughout the day.

Here's why sucrose is so important: First, this disaccharide is made up of glucose and fructose. The glucose is used for immediate energy, and the body sends the fructose to the liver either to be converted into glucose for more immediate energy (if it's needed right then) or, more likely, it goes into storage as glycogen for use later on. This means that only half of the sucrose you eat becomes readily available energy, glucose.

When you compare the digestion of sugar to the digestion of a starch such as bread, you come to an astonishing conclusion: You get more quick energy from the *starch* in foods than you do from the *sugar* in foods. Why? Because starch breaks down into maltose, 100 percent of which becomes glucose, but only 50 percent of sucrose gets converted into glucose. Hold that thought for a little later on when I discuss how different kinds of carbs—both starches and sugars—affect blood-glucose levels and your health in general.

✔ **Food Fact**: On average, Americans are currently consuming somewhere between 20 and 31 teaspoons of added sugar a day. That comes to 300 to 500 extra calories!

✔ **Food Fact**: The USDA suggests limiting the amount of added sugars based on total daily calories:

6 teaspoons/day for 1,600 calories
12 teasoons for 2,200 calories
18 teaspoons for 2,800 calories
To translate:
 6 tsp. sugar = 1 cup ice cream
 12 tsp. sugar = 12 oz. fruit drink or flavored tea
 18 tsp. sugar = 2 cans Coke or Pepsi

Table Sugar 101

What is table sugar made from? Sucrose is actually refined sugar cane or sugar-beet juice that gets processed into granules (granulated sugar).

See pages 114–118 for explanations about high-fructose corn syrup, sugar alcohols, and other sweeteners.

The Disaccharides: Lactose

Lactose, the sugar found in milk, is also a disaccharide that breaks down into glucose and galactose. The glucose part of lactose provides you with an immediate energy source, while the liver handles the galactose (much as it does with the fructose in sucrose). Lactose gives some people stomach trouble: Lactose-intolerant people have lower levels of the enzyme that breaks down this sugar in their intestines. When lactose sits in the gut and is poorly digested, it ferments, creating cramps, bloating, gas, and diarrhea. If this annoying and uncomfortable problem affects you, you may want to consume: (1) only small amounts of the offending foods, (2) lactose-reduced or lactose-free milk products, or (3) lactase capsules when you eat dairy foods.

✔ **Food Fact:** Lactose intolerance is not the same as a milk allergy, which is caused by a person's immune reaction to the protein in milk.

Double Sugars (Disaccharides)

	Breaks down into	Purpose	Found in
Maltose	glucose + glucose	Used for immediate energy	Any starchy food
Sucrose	glucose + fructose	Used for immediate and stored energy	Table sugar
Lactose	glucose + galactose	Used for immediate and stored energy	All forms of milk and milk products

The Complex Carbohydrates

Some carbs are complex because they are structurally much larger molecules than the simple carbs; they consist of many glucose units attached together, known chemically as a *polysaccharide*. The complex carbs consist of *glycogen* (how animals, including humans, store unused glucose), *starch* (how plants store unused glucose), and the *fibers* found in plant foods. Animals use their glycogen stores when the glucose supply is low; plants do the same thing with their starch reserves.

The Polysaccharides: Glycogen

Here's everything you need to know about glycogen: It's a complex carbohydrate found in your body but *not* in the food you eat. Fructose and galactose molecules resulting from carbohydrate digestion go to the liver, where they are stored in a form that you can use later for quick energy.

By the way, your liver also gives unused glucose molecules this same treatment: It turns glucose into glycogen and stores it right there in the liver or in muscle cells. Your body can use your liver's glycogen for immediate energy if it's needed to supplement a low glucose supply, such as during the night; but the muscles' glycogen usually sticks around to be used within the muscle cells. Because glycogen is made up of many glucose molecules, when you need energy from either your liver or your muscles, the molecules easily break apart the bonds holding the glucoses together. The result? A surge of energy. And here we are, back to glucose again, and back to your body's retrieving glucose from its favorite fuel source, carbohydrates (in this particular case, glycogen).

Your Glycogen Stores

Your body collects a reserve of an easily broken-down starch supply called glycogen, which is stored in the liver and in muscle cells. The liver's glycogen stores add to the supply of energy to your brain, nerve cells, and other organs when your blood-glucose levels are low. The muscles' glycogen stores are used by the muscles themselves. And remember: Your body dips into these supplies *only* when blood-glucose levels are inadequate for its immediate energy needs.

The Polysaccharides: Plant Starch

Starch is to plants what glycogen is to humans: glucose in a stored form. There can be hundreds, even thousands, of glucose molecules linked together to form a starch molecule, so they really are "big guys" in the molecule world. Plants such as yams or grains of rice store their energy—their glucose—as starch to use as needed for growth.

Luckily for us humans, we can digest most plant starches. Just think of all the times you've eaten wheat, corn, rice, and potatoes! Starches prevail in our food supply, and your body knows how to break them down to get the fuel it needs—glucose.

✔ **Food Fact:** A 1-inch cube of a starchy food such as potatoes may contain as many as one million starch molecules.

The Polysaccharides: Plant Fibers

The fibers in plants are essential to their survival. These fibers support the plant and transport oxygen, water, and nutrients to all of its parts. We get dietary plant fibers from every plant we eat, whether it's a fruit or a vegetable, a grain or a legume, as long as the fibers haven't been removed during some refining process.

Like the other complex carbohydrates glycogen and starch, plant fibers are also polysaccharides; that is, they're also made up of many sugar molecules linked together. But there's a difference between the other polysaccharides and plant starches: Your body can't digest them at all. (To tell the truth, some fibers can be digested by some of the *bacteria* that live in the human gut but not by your body itself.) For this reason, plant fibers are defined as non-starch polysaccharides, or "unavailable" carbohydrates. (In contrast, all sugars, as well as glycogen and starch, represent your body's available sources of carbohydrates.) But don't think unkindly of fibers, because they still play an important role. Simply because they remain virtually intact in the gut, they help to lower blood cholesterol and slow down food digestion and glucose absorption (which is good for you, as I'll explain later). They also increase the bulk in your stool.

There are about seven different types of fibers important in your diet, and a few of them may even sound familiar: You may have come across these polysaccharides while following a high-fiber or weight-loss diet. You may also have seen fiber listed as an ingredient on many food labels.

Soluble Fiber

Four of the fibers are *soluble*: *pectins, gums, mucilages,* and some *hemicelluloses.* Your body's intestinal bacteria can digest these fibers, and as they do, the fibers break down into a gel. This gel does a host of wonderful things, such as lower cholesterol and regulate blood-glucose levels for long periods of time. You'll find soluble fibers in plant foods such as oat and rice brans, rolled oats, barley, beans, carrots, and unpeeled apples, among others.

Where's the Fiber?

True or False? Foods derived from animal sources (meats, eggs, cheese, and milk, for example) contain no fiber.
Answer: True.

Insoluble Fiber

There are three types of *insoluble* fibers: *cellulose,* many *hemicelluloses,* and *lignans.* These fibers can absorb large amounts of water in the digestive tract, so they make up the bulk that you eventually eliminate. Here are some of the great things insoluble fibers do for you. They:

- decrease appetite
- slow the rate that your blood takes in the glucose that is formed from digested sugars and starches
- improve, or even cure, constipation
- decrease your risk of hemorrhoids, diverticulosis, and irritable bowel syndrome

Wheat bran (found in whole-grain cereals, breads, and crackers) is the richest source of insoluble dietary fiber. Other sources include legumes such as kidney, pinto, and lima beans.

Even though most of the fibers you eat don't produce glucose, they still affect how fast glucose gets dumped into your bloodstream. So even these carbs play an influential role in our day-to-day lives and overall good health. But there's still much more to the story.

Complex Carbohydrates (Polysaccharides)

	Purpose	Found in
Glycogen	Used for quick-release from stored energy	No foods contain glycogen; stored in muscle cells and the liver
Starch	Used for immediate energy	Wheat, corn, rice, potatoes, etc.
Plant Fibers	Decrease appetite, slow the rate of glucose absorption, ease constipation	**Soluble:** oat and rice brans, rolled oats, barley, beans, carrots, unpeeled apples
	Reduce risk of hemorrhoids, diverticulosis, and irritable bowel syndrome	**Insoluble:** wheat bran, legumes, fruits, vegetables

Why Are Carbohydrates So Important?

> ➤ Your body likes to get energy from carbohydrates; that's why carbs are your body's fuel of choice.

> ➤ Glucose is the energy form your body uses for all its activities.

> ➤ If you eat a balanced diet, at least half of your daily calories come from carbohydrates, so you're giving your body a majority of calories it will use for its energy needs throughout the day and night, in the form it prefers.

Name That Sugar

Here are some common forms of sugar that you might find on a food's Nutrition Facts label:

- ➤ brown sugar
- ➤ cane sugar
- ➤ confectioners' sugar
- ➤ corn syrup
- ➤ crystallized cane sugar
- ➤ dextrin
- ➤ dextrose
- ➤ evaporated cane juice
- ➤ fruit juice concentrate
- ➤ high-fructose corn syrup
- ➤ honey
- ➤ invert sugar
- ➤ malt
- ➤ maltodextrin
- ➤ maple syrup
- ➤ molasses
- ➤ raw sugar
- ➤ turbinado sugar

Carbohydrate Digestion and Absorption

Question: Why does your body digest food?

Answer: To get the energy it needs to carry out all of its daily activities.

Question: What form of energy does your body use?
Answer: Glucose.

Question: Which are the easiest foods for your body to digest into glucose?
Answer: Carbohydrates.

Question: Why?
Answer: Because glucose is *already* a carbohydrate; your body doesn't have to work very hard to get energy from it. It likes that. That's why your body treats carbs preferentially.

Question: How does your body get the glucose and deliver it into the blood?
Answer: Keep reading!

Carb Digestion

To help illustrate the digestive process, let's follow the path of a piece of bread as it moves through your digestive system, starting with your mouth.

- With the help of your tongue, your teeth grind, tear, and pull the bread apart. Meanwhile, your saliva covers the bread.
- Amylase, a digestive enzyme in your saliva, begins breaking apart some of those huge starch molecules into shorter and shorter polysaccharides and eventually splits some of them into disaccharide maltose molecules. (Remember the experiment of holding a piece of bread in your mouth long enough to taste the sweetness of the maltose molecules?) This is a time-sensitive process, because food doesn't stay in your mouth for long.
- Once you swallow it, the bread travels down the esophagus and after a few minutes enters your stomach. The stomach works a little bit like a washing machine, bathing the bread in hydrochloric acid and gastric enzymes.

▶ When the "cycle" is finished, your stomach's acids have disinfected the bread. (And it's a good thing too: Consider all the bacteria you eat when you put food into your mouth.) In addition: (1) your body has digested the enzyme amylase that attached to the bread in your mouth, so its digestive role is over; (2) the hydrochloric acid splits whatever disaccharides have formed so far, mainly maltose into glucose; (3) more polysaccharides are breaking down into more disaccharides; and (4) any fibers in the bread have unraveled from the starch but remain undigested and linger in your stomach. This lingering slows down the movement of the just-formed simple carbohydrates into the small intestine.

▶ The next stop inside the digestive tract is the small intestine, a 20-plus-foot-long tube, the Grand Central Station of the whole digestive process. It's in the small intestine where most of the bread will be completely broken down.

▶ All of the starch molecules have by now become maltose molecules and then glucose molecules.

▶ The small intestine is the end of the line for just about all of the bread's digestion; the fiber in the bread will move down into the large intestine and be eliminated.

▶ The result of digestion: glucose; and possibly fructose and galactose if any ingredients, such as milk or sugar, have been added to the bread before baking.

Just as a reminder: I'm describing carbohydrate digestion because this is a book about carbs. Your body also digests dietary proteins and fats, as I explained earlier (see page 7).

Carb Absorption

To sum up: During digestion, your body breaks down carbs into the form of energy it can most immediately use, glucose, which is transferred from the intestinal cells into the blood. Your blood carries it throughout your body by *absorption*.

▶ Because of specialized cells on its lining, your small intestine is perfectly suited to transfer glucose out of the gut and into your bloodstream. These cells, called *villi*, look like tiny fingerlike projections.

▶ The villi allow glucose to leave the intestinal wall and get carried away by the circulating blood.

▶ The blood flows straight to and through the liver, where all of the monosaccharides (glucose and possibly fructose and galactose) are processed.

▶ The result of absorption: Glucose exits the liver and moves into the circulating blood and is ready for use.

So, to repeat:

Question: How does your body actually get the glucose from carbohydrate foods and deliver it into the blood?

Answer: It digests the food that has been eaten by passing it through the digestive organs (mouth, esophagus, stomach, small intestine, and liver) breaking it down further and further until it consists of just the single sugar glucose, which passes from the liver and into the bloodstream.

Glucose in Your Body and in Your Blood

Whew! That's a lot of work for your body to do, and it does the job every time you eat. But the job description isn't quite complete: What goes on once the glucose is finally circulating throughout your body? How do you extract energy from the glucose molecule?

First, the glucose molecule has to get *inside* the cell that needs the energy. I'll go into more detail about this process in a later chapter, but for now, the simple explanation is that a carrier (insulin) escorts the glucose into the cell.

▶ Once the glucose is inside the cell, many complicated chemical reactions have to occur in a certain sequence in order for it to produce the energy you need.

▶ Enzymes break the glucose molecule in half; these halves can be put back together again or they can be further broken down into smaller segments.

▶ Because the smaller segments can't be reassembled back into glucose, one of two things will happen to them: (1) they can be either turned into body fat; or (2) they can be completely broken down into three end products: carbon dioxide, water and . . . *energy.*

▶ As long as there's a constant supply of dietary carbs available, this process hums along with minimal effort. Remember, your body is just following its instincts to turn carbs into energy.

▶ While you are digesting carbs into glucose for immediate energy, you are also digesting proteins into amino acids to meet your protein needs, and fats into fatty acids to store in your energy reserves. Insulin helps make all of these deliveries; its escort service allows your cells to receive the simplest digestive products: glucose, amino acids, and fatty acids.

So that is it, in a pretty big nutshell! The explanation above shows why carbohydrates are your body's fuel of choice and why your body wants to use carbs above all other nutrients for glucose, its energy source.

What's Insulin, Anyway?

What is insulin?	A hormone.
Where is it made?	In your pancreas.
What does it do?	Controls the transport of glucose, amino acids, and fatty acids from the bloodstream into your cells.

THE BOTTOM LINE

➤ All living cells need energy.

➤ The six simple carbohydrates are glucose, fructose, galactose, maltose, sucrose, and lactose.

➤ The three complex carbohydrates are glycogen, plant starch, and the plant fibers.

➤ Your body digests food by passing it through your digestive organs, breaking it down until it consists of simple sugars, amino acids, and fatty acids.

➤ Insulin escorts glucose, amino acids, and fatty acids into the cells where they're used.

➤ Glucose, which results from the breaking down of carbohydrates, is the form of energy used by the body to carry out its daily activities and functions.

3

GUSHERS AND TRICKLERS: AN INTRODUCTION

A quick recap: Your body ingests food. In a balanced diet the majority of these food calories come from carbohydrates. And then your body digests this food for energy to do its daily work. The energy from these carbs takes a form called glucose, your body's preferred food source.

Digesting food is a multi-step process, which, most of the time starts and finishes without your awareness that it's even going on. Once digestion is complete, the final products are properly packaged away: Amino acids (from protein digestion) head into cells so they can repair, replace, and maintain the health of organs and muscles; fatty acids (from fat digestion) move into cells as a form of stored energy; and the just-formed glucose molecules from carbohydrate digestion get packaged away too—into the bloodstream as the energy you will start using right away.

In order for glucose to be useful, though, it must get *inside* the cells. And, as I briefly mentioned in the last chapter, this is where that metabolic megastar, insulin, enters the picture. Here is how cells get "zapped" with energy:

- When glucose enters the bloodstream after digestion, it meets up with other glucose molecules already there. (The blood always contains some glucose.) Your brain starts a series of reactions that will eventually move the glucose out of your blood and into the cells, where it needs to be.
- Your brain activates the pancreas to secrete insulin. Why? Because the glucose can't move itself from the

blood into the cells—it needs to be carried, and insulin is the carrier.

▶ Under normal conditions, the appropriate amount of insulin that your body needs for the actual glucose load (also called "glycemic load") at that time is the amount that your pancreas secretes into the blood.

▶ An insulin molecule picks up a glucose molecule and escorts it over to a cell. On the membrane of the cell there are several receptor sites; let's call them "doors." Insulin has the "key" to open the "door." Now the glucose molecule can enter the cell and give it the energy it needs to do the work it is supposed to do.

▶ As this process continues over time, more and more glucose gets moved into more and more cells and now you've got one pumped-up body that has the energy it needs to carry out its functions, day or night.

▶ After about four to five hours, your blood-glucose level starts to drop again, because for several hours, glucose has been moving out of your blood and into your cells nonstop. So, if you are awake, you eat, and the process starts all over again.

This summarizes what happens under normal circumstances in a healthy body, that is, a body without diabetes or glucose intolerance.

The Pancreas Profile

The pancreas is a soft grayish-white gland that rests behind the stomach, is about eight inches long, and weighs just two or three ounces. It's about the size of a small, thick checkbook or a pencil case. This gland provides several of the enzymes you need to digest food into energy; it also makes hormones that help your body use that energy. The pancreas is the only place in your whole body that makes that ever-famous glucose-escort hormone, insulin. And it's only a certain kind of cell in the pancreas, the beta cell, that produces insulin. The special role that the beta cells in the pancreas play makes them critical to good health. If, for some reason, the beta cells can't produce insulin, the glucose that has entered the blood after digestion has nowhere to go, so it stays in the blood. Too much glucose can lead to elevated blood sugars, which may result in diabetes.

> **Did You Know . . .** that your pancreas changes from grayish-white to a rosy pink when it's secreting insulin?

The Beta Business

Beta cells make and secrete insulin. In fact, these cells make insulin all the time, but if you haven't eaten, their activity is minimal. Once the food you eat enters your gut and digestion starts to elevate blood-glucose levels, the beta cells are stimulated to step up their insulin production. At first—a minute or two after you eat—stored insulin in the pancreas shoots out into the blood. In the meantime, the beta cells start working full force and continue to secrete insulin as it is needed. Usually the resting (or "basal") level of insulin secretion returns within three hours after you've eaten your meal or snack.

✔ **Fun Fact:** There are millions of beta cells in the pancreas.

> **Did You Know . . .** that a healthy pancreas secretes 20 to 30 units of insulin every day?

"Gushers" vs. "Tricklers"

How well your body functions at specific times throughout the day or night depends on how quickly it makes glucose available to expectant cells—the difference between "gusher" foods and "trickler" foods. For example, sometimes you need a surge of energy (from a gusher) because your blood-glucose level is low; orange juice will do a better job of quickly raising the sugar level than an egg and cheese sandwich or a milk shake. At other times, you're looking for a steady stream of a more constant flow of energy (from a trickler), such as when you're taking a three-hour hike or wallpapering a room. Then, a bowl of rolled oats with milk and peaches will provide this kind of sustained energy better than a sleeve of salty crackers or some rice cakes with jelly. That's the difference between gushers and tricklers. (See the chart below for an illustration of how tricklers offer a steady release of energy compared to gushers.)

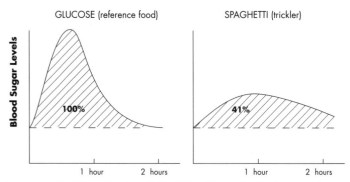

Adapted from *The Glucose Revolution Pocket Guide to Diabetes.* Reprinted courtesy of Marlowe & Company.

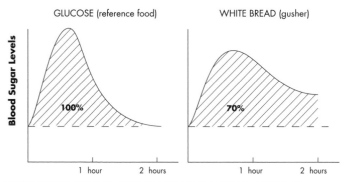

Adapted from *The Glucose Revolution.* Reprinted courtesy of Marlowe & Company.

	Gushers	**Tricklers**
What types of food?	Quickly digested carbohydrates	Slowly digested carbohydrates
Why are the foods digested this way? (See page 135 for list of factors influencing rate of digestion.)	Because of the major ingredient in a food (such as enriched wheat flour in white bread) or because of the extensive processing methods used to manufacture a food (like puffing up Rice Krispies or rice cakes), your body has a quick and easy time of breaking down the carb molecules into glucose, allowing for rapid digestion.	Because of the major ingredient in a food (such as 100% stoneground whole wheat flour in whole-grain bread) or because of the minimal processing (such as in rolled oats rather than instant oats), your body has much more work to do to break the carb molecules into glucose; they will all be digested, but the process will take much longer to complete.
How does digestion happen?	Once the glucose molecules are readied in the small intestine, they exit into the blood. If many molecules are ready at the same time, they will all leave at the same time and "gush" into the blood, creating a surge, or spike, of blood glucose.	If the starch molecules in, say, a slice of 100% whole wheat bread are protected by several layers of fibrous tissue (bran), or if they are compressed into a tiny dense product such as Bran Buds, the digestive enzymes have a lot of breakdown work to do. It's as though the starch molecules are on a slow-moving conveyor belt going through the small intestine, where, at each station a little more, and then a little more, of the starch gets broken down. When a glucose molecule is finally produced, it hops off the conveyor belt and into the blood. This process produces a more constant, even flow (a "trickle") of energy for a longer period of time.
Examples	Cornflakes, sticky rice, rice cakes, dates, Gatorade, instant oatmeal	Bran, al dente pasta, yams, milk, lentils, old-fashioned oats, apples

The Roller-Coaster Effects of Gushers

In a glucose-tolerant, nondiabetic person, if blood-glucose levels gush up because of eating many quickly digested carbohydrate calories, they're going to come crashing down. (Review: This is because your body meets the high glucose load with a huge outpouring of insulin from the pancreas and also because the cells are sensitive to insulin's presence and open up to let the glucose inside them.) So, as a result, first there's a lot of glucose in the blood, and then there's a lot less, because now it has moved into the cells.

This rapid rise—then drop—in glucose levels can make you feel hungry, tired, shaky, headachy, unfocused, and irritable—the classic signs of low blood sugar (also called *hypoglycemia*). It's interesting to note that these are also the classic symptoms that many chronic dieters experience.

hypo = low
glyc = sugar
emia = blood

If you have type 2 diabetes, gushers bring blood-glucose levels up, and then your body has a difficult time lowering those levels again. (Another review: This is due to insufficient insulin and/or the lack of cooperation from the cells to allow the glucose to enter them.)

If you don't have diabetes, a steady diet of gushers makes you hungry, tired, and irritable. And here's another unfriendly effect that gushers can have—in people with or without diabetes: They encourage your body to store fat. How do gushers lead to fat storage? Because gusher calories force more insulin to circulate in the blood, and the more insulin moving around in the blood, the greater the likelihood that some glucose as well as fatty acids, in the form of triglycerides, will be put away into storage as fat.

Cruise Control with Tricklers

By their very definition, slowly digested carbs, or tricklers, don't give blood-glucose levels much of a roller-coaster ride. Tricklers provide a more steady, even energy flow into the blood and promote a more constant flow of energy out of the blood and into the cells. It's like driving a car in cruise control; with little effort, a steady, even flow of fuel passes through the motor and keeps the car running smoothly until it is time for another fill-up.

Your body performs as well as the car when its energy (or fuel) supply is constant: You have the right amount of energy to draw from for your daily activities, those you deliberately perform, such as climbing stairs or working at a computer, as well as those activities that you perform without realizing it, such as breathing and digesting your breakfast. With adequate energy, your body feels in control of its energy supply; it knows it won't run dry and can make it to the next fill-up. In fact, slowly digested carbs can help you avoid that tongue-hanging exhaustion at the end of the day. Slowly digested calories from trickler carbs in a well-balanced lunch provide you with a sense of fullness until you can prepare and eat dinner at night. This constant energy supply will not only keep you feeling satisfied from meal to meal, it will also help you to make better, controlled food choices—not impulsive ones that result from feeling ravenously hungry, tired, and hypoglycemic.

As if these benefits of tricklers were not enough, there's another bonus to eating them: They discourage your body from storing fat by encouraging it to use the available glucose for immediate energy. Eat a well-balanced diet, which includes "trickler" carbs in adequate, not excessive, amounts, and lose weight. Not exactly a magic bullet, but certainly easy enough to do. (There is more about the weight-loss advantages of trickler carbs later, in chapter 5.)

The Gusher/Trickler Identification Profile

You can tell whether a food is a gusher or a trickler by . . .

▶ How much a starch swells up when it's cooked
Gushers: A lot
    Examples: Sticky rice, overcooked pasta
Tricklers: Minimal
    Examples: Long-grain rice, brown rice, al dente
    pasta
▶ How fibrous the food is
Gushers: Low fiber content
    Examples: Bagels, hard rolls, cornflakes
Tricklers: High fiber content
    Examples: Whole-grain breads, All-Bran, lentils,
    barley
▶ How much processing the food has undergone (pumping in air, refining, or milling of whole grains)
Gushers: Significant
    Examples: Rice cakes, instant oatmeal, enriched
    wheat breads
Tricklers: Minimal
    Examples: Old-fashioned or rolled oats, 100%
    whole wheat bread
▶ How acidic the food is
Gushers: Low or slight acid content
    Examples: Angel food cake
Tricklers: High acid content
    Examples: Sourdough bread products
▶ How sweet the food is
Gushers: A lot of sugar, with little or minimal fiber,
    protein, or fat
    Examples: Gatorade, sugar wafers
Tricklers: Some sugar, also containing some fiber,
    protein, or fat
    Examples: Social Tea biscuits, shortbread, arrowroot cookies, peanut M&Ms

How to Calculate a Mixed Meal

Keep in mind that when eaten *alone,* gusher foods will cause their signature glucose spike and, when eaten *alone,* tricklers cause a longer-lasting supply of sugar in the blood. But what happens when we eat a meal that has a *mix* of gushers and tricklers? Well, first remember that the glucose is coming from the *carbohydrates* in your meal, so you want to look at those foods—which types and how much of them you ate. Consider how much a part of the entire carb intake each carbohydrate food contributes (is it 10 percent of all the carbs in the meal, or 50 percent). When you add it all up, if there are more gusher calories being digested from the meal, you'll experience a more rapid rise in blood glucose than if you had eaten more trickler calories. (The presence of proteins and fats in the meal will also influence glucose levels, but that is in the next chapter.)

THE BOTTOM LINE

➤ Gushers, or quickly digested carbs, create blood-glucose spikes that leave you feeling hungry, tired, and irritable. They encourage fat storage.

➤ Tricklers, or slowly digested carbs, keep your blood-glucose levels on an even keel, so you feel energized and full. They discourage fat storage.

➤ How quickly your body digests a carbohydrate depends on several factors, for example, its ingredients and its processing and preparation.

4

THE GLYCEMIC INDEX: A WAY TO RANK CARBS

Why is it that we know so much about gushers and tricklers? The differing effects of quickly digested and slowly digested carbohydrates on blood-glucose levels are now common knowledge thanks to the unrelenting efforts of several researchers who understood what was happening in carbohydrate digestion and sought to prove it scientifically.

In 1981 scientists in Toronto were researching which foods were best for people with diabetes. Up to that time, people with diabetes were given dietary exchanges to follow, that is, certain foods in certain portions could be substituted or exchanged for other nutritionally similar foods. So, for example, a half cup of mashed potatoes could easily be "exchanged" in a meal for a half cup of pasta. The presumption was that these two starches would produce the same blood-glucose response once they were digested, and that the response would be a slow, modest rise of glucose into the blood. And the other piece of advice given to people with diabetes was that they should avoid sugar and not be too concerned about bread, rice, potatoes, and so on, since these were starchy (not sweet) carbs and, therefore, would not produce high rises in glucose levels.

When these ideas were actually put to the test in the Toronto labs, scientists made an astonishing discovery: The investigators found, for example, that fruits such as apples or grapes, despite their sugar content, caused blood sugars to rise less than plain sliced white bread! But how could that be? Weren't sugars supposed to raise blood-glucose and weren't starches supposed to have less effect on blood-glucose?

That wasn't what the researchers found: Their laboratory tests proved that some *foods with sugar did not produce the expected high, rapid rise in blood-glucose levels, while some starchy foods did.* In other words, the new dietary message for people with diabetes was that some starches elevate blood-glucose as much as, or even more than, some sweet or sugary foods. This research gave birth to the glycemic index (GI), what I informally call the "gushers" and "tricklers."

The glycemic index is a ranking of carbohydrates based on their immediate effect on blood-glucose levels. All tested foods are compared with a reference food, such as pure glucose. (See illustration on page 31.) The ranking is based on a scale of 0 to 100. Glucose has a GI value of 100 because it doesn't have to break down any further. The more quickly a carbohydrate breaks down into glucose, the closer its GI value is to 100. And the more slowly a carb becomes glucose, the lower its GI value.

The Research Continues

Scientists around the world continue to test carbohydrate foods for their glycemic index values. In fact, to date, researchers have tested more than 600 commonly eaten carbohydrates. Clinical studies throughout the world continue to prove that the glycemic index is a valid tool for blood-glucose control. You can find more detailed information about the glycemic index at the following Web sites:

- www.glycemicindex.com
- www.mendosa.com/gi.htm
- www.fifty50.com
- www.health.harvard.edu/article.cfm?id=48

Part 2 of this book illustrates specific health advantages of choosing low-GI foods over high-GI foods when you eat them as part of a balanced diet. Some of those benefits include blood-glucose control, weight management, heart health, athletic performance, and endurance. But the best side effect from a low-GI diet is how good it makes you feel!

Did You Know . . . that "glycemic" means "sugar" + "in blood"?

The Glycemic Index: What's In, What's Out

Which foods will you find listed in the glycemic index?
Carbohydrates.
Which foods won't you find listed in the glycemic index?
Most proteins and fats.

Brain Teaser #1:

Why are *mostly* carbohydrate foods listed in the glycemic index?

➤ Which foods are your body's fuel of choice?
Carbohydrates.
➤ In a balanced diet, which foods contribute the most calories to be used for energy? *Carbohydrates.*
➤ Which, of all the foods you eat, most affects blood-sugar levels? *Carbohydrates.*
➤ If the glycemic index focuses on those foods that most affect blood-glucose levels, which foods would it be looking at? *Carbohydrates.*

Now you know which foods are listed in the glycemic index and why.

Brain Teaser #2:

High-protein foods and fats *aren't* listed in the glycemic index. Why not?

➤ Which, of all the foods you eat, most affects blood-sugar levels? *Carbohydrates.*
➤ Which, of all the foods you eat, least affects blood-sugar levels? *Proteins and fats.*
➤ Why don't protein foods affect blood-glucose levels? *Because the majority of protein calories are used to restore and rebuild the many different body cells; they're not normally converted into glucose for immediate energy.*

➤ Why don't fats affect blood-glucose levels? *Because your body puts 95 percent of fats into storage for future, rather than immediate, energy use.*

➤ What's the purpose of the glycemic index? *To rank those foods that affect blood-glucose levels.*

➤ Which foods most affect blood-glucose levels? *Carbohydrates.*

➤ Which foods does the glycemic index rank? *Carbohydrates.*

Now you know which foods are not listed in the glycemic index and why.

Note: Exceptions to the protein and fat rule include milk and yogurt, and legumes such as lentils and chickpeas. These foods are high in protein (and sometimes fat) but they also have a high carbohydrate content, which is why they've been tested and included in the glycemic index.

The Glycemic Index at Your Table

Does the glycemic index apply to meals as it does to individual carbs? What happens when we eat a meal that contains many foods, including gushers *and* tricklers? First keep in mind that your after-meal blood-glucose level, your glycemic load, is coming from the carbs you've eaten—which types and how much of them. And then, the presence of proteins, fats, fiber, and acidic foods and other factors will also influence how quickly glucose gets into your bloodstream. Can you imagine: your body takes all of this into account before blood-sugar levels rise after a meal?

If you eat an average portion of a high-GI food, will your blood-glucose level spike? You know the answer is yes. But what if you eat a *large* portion of a *low*-GI food, will your blood-glucose level also spike? The answer, again, is yes! The amount of glucose streaming into your blood from your gut has to do with the *quality* of the carb (its GI value) and it has to do with the *quantity* of the carb (its GL, or glycemic load). Compare converted white rice to sticky rice:

½ cup converted white rice (22g carbs)	GI = 38 (low)	GL = 8 (low)
½ cup sticky rice (29g carbs)	GI = 98 (high)	GL = 28 (high)

What these numbers show is that there are more than three times as many glucose molecules entering your blood from the sticky rice (GL is 28) as from the same amount of converted white rice (GL is 8). And so it's good to remember that if you want to enjoy some sticky rice, just have a little bit to prevent your blood-glucose level from spiking. This illustrates to you how a food's GI value (its *quality*) impacts on your blood-glucose levels.

Now let's look at how the glycemic load of a food (its *quantity*) also affects blood-glucose levels. If you eat 1½ cups of converted white rice instead of ½ cup, what happens? Keep in mind that converted white rice is a slowly digested carb.

½ cup converted white rice (22g carbs)	GI = 38 (low)	GL = 8 (low)
1½ cups converted white rice (66g carbs)	GI = 38 (low)	GL = 24 (high)

What this means is that, by eating 1½ cups of the rice, your bloodstream has to deal with an overload of glucose molecules, not because you ate a gusher carb, but simply because you ate *too much of a trickler!* This is why I harp so much about portion sizes with my patients.

If you are tempted to figure out the glycemic loads of the portions that you eat of your favorite carbs, here's how you do it:

Glycemic Load = (grams carbohydrate in your serving x GI of the food) ÷ 100

Low GL	=	0–10
Moderate GL	=	11–19
High GL	=	20 or more

What should the glycemic load be for a whole day?

Low = less than 80
High = more than 120

Rating the Glycemic Index of Foods

Food	G. I. Value
High GI (gusher)	70 or greater
Moderate GI	56–69
Low GI (trickler)	0–55

High-GI Foods

▶ Instant mashed potatoes (97)
▶ Cornflakes (92)
▶ Gatorade (89)
▶ Pretzels (83)
▶ Rice cakes (82)
▶ Watermelon (72)
▶ Popcorn (72)

Moderate-GI Foods

▶ Pancakes (from mix) (67)
▶ Stoned Wheat Thins (67)
▶ Cantaloupe (65)
▶ Raisins (64)
▶ Hamburger bun (61)
▶ Cheese pizza (60)
▶ Mini Wheats (58)

Low-GI Foods

▶ Potato chips (54)
▶ Light ice cream (50)
▶ Carrots (47)
▶ Rolled oats (42)

- Spaghetti (al dente) (38)
- Skim milk (32)
- Cherries (22)

So what's so great about the glycemic index? It illustrates how blood-glucose levels are affected by how quickly or how slowly you digest carbohydrates. The glycemic index spells it all out for you: Foods with a high GI value are gushers, while foods with a low GI value are tricklers. In the appendix of this book, I've categorized a long list of carbohydrate foods into three categories that can help you make clear choices in your daily diet with regard to carbohydrate *quality*. By keeping your eye on portion size you will also address your glycemic load; that is your carbohydrate *quantity*.

THE BOTTOM LINE

➤ Some starches elevate blood sugars as much as, or even more than, some sugary or sweet foods.

➤ The glycemic index ranks carbohydrates based on their immediate effect on blood-glucose levels.

➤ Tricklers are foods with a low glycemic index value.

➤ Gushers are foods with a high glycemic index value.

➤ Glycemic load helps you predict how your blood-glucose level will respond to a specific amount of a specific carbohydrate food once it has been consumed.

Good Carbs: Your Edge Against Disease

5

EAT GOOD CARBS,
LOSE WEIGHT

If you live in Colorado, the thinnest state in America, you may not have a weight problem. The same may be true if you live in the northeastern states of Massachusetts, Vermont, Connecticut, or Rhode Island. Overall, these states have the fewest obese adults. But for the majority of states, the adult obesity rate is more than 20 percent, with West Virginia topping the list at 28 percent.

Our national obsession with weight loss continues to thrive, but, perhaps more in thought than in deed. According to one recent survey, although nearly six out of ten American adults realize they need to lose weight, the majority of these people admit to inadequate regular exercise and consuming too many calories most, if not all, days.

So there are no surprises in the following statistics:

- 127 million adults in the U.S. are overweight, 60 million are obese, and 9 million are severely obese.
- In just over ten years, the prevalence of obesity in the U.S. has increased by more than *70 percent.*
- According to the Centers for Disease Control and Prevention, there are *no government statistics for the prevalence of severe obesity prior to 1988.*
- At least 15 percent of American children (ages 6 to 19) are overweight.
- The cost to treat obesity-related health problems was approximately *$117 billion* in 2000.

These are sobering numbers that point to the extent of the problem. What terms define the various degrees of severity of the problem. Are you considered overweight? Are you obese, and, if so, how severely?

Overweight or Obese or What?

Of course you know whether or not you're gaining extra weight: your clothes feel tighter, it's harder to bend over to tie your shoes, or that bus or plane seat feels snugger than on the last trip. No matter what the sign, you don't need someone else—your doctor, your spouse, or your best friend—to tell you. No one knows better than you do. Sure, you could think that you're overweight and not be. That's also a medical problem, but not our focus right now. For most of us, if we think we're overweight, we probably are. But let's not be judgmental; let's go with the facts. First, let me clarify some terms.

> **Did You Know . . .** that obesity is the second leading cause of *preventable* death in the U.S.? 400,000 deaths result from poor diet and physical inactivity. (Only smoking kills more people—435,000 in 2000.)

Determine Your Body Mass Index (BMI)

Measuring your BMI is the most popular way to determine whether you're overweight. This measurement shows the relationship of your weight to your height. Check the table on page 49 for your BMI to identify your weight status classification. If you want to calculate your BMI for yourself, here's the formula:

$$\text{BMI} = \frac{\text{weight in pounds} \times 703}{(\text{height in inches}) \times (\text{height in inches})}$$

Example: Let's say that you're 5′9″ and weigh 250 pounds. Here's how you would calculate your BMI:

250 lbs. x 703 ÷ 69 in. x 69 in. = 175,750 = 37 (BMI)

Body Mass Index Table

BMI	19	20	21	22	23	24	25	26	27	28	29	30	31	32	33	34	35	36	37	38	39	40	41	42	43	44	45	46	47	48	49	50	51	52	53	54
	Normal						Overweight					Obese										Extreme Obesity														
Height (inches)												Body Weight (pounds)																								
58	91	96	100	105	110	115	119	124	129	134	138	143	148	153	158	162	167	172	177	181	186	191	196	201	205	210	215	220	224	229	234	239	244	248	253	258
59	94	99	104	109	114	119	124	128	133	138	143	148	153	158	163	168	173	178	183	188	193	198	203	208	212	217	222	227	232	237	242	247	252	257	262	267
60	97	102	107	112	118	123	128	133	138	143	148	153	158	163	168	174	179	184	189	194	199	204	209	215	220	225	230	235	240	245	250	255	261	266	271	276
61	100	106	111	116	122	127	132	137	143	148	153	158	164	169	174	180	185	190	195	201	206	211	217	222	227	232	238	243	248	254	259	264	269	275	280	285
62	104	109	115	120	126	131	136	142	147	153	158	164	169	175	180	186	191	196	202	207	213	218	224	229	235	240	246	251	256	262	267	273	278	284	289	295
63	107	113	118	124	130	135	141	146	152	158	163	169	175	180	186	191	197	203	208	214	220	225	231	237	242	248	254	259	265	270	278	282	287	293	299	304
64	110	116	122	128	134	140	145	151	157	163	169	174	180	186	192	197	204	209	216	222	228	232	238	244	250	256	262	267	273	279	285	291	296	302	308	314
65	114	120	126	132	138	144	150	156	162	168	174	180	186	192	198	204	210	216	222	228	234	240	246	252	258	264	270	276	282	288	294	300	306	312	318	324
66	118	124	130	136	142	148	155	161	167	173	179	186	192	198	204	210	216	223	229	235	241	247	253	260	266	272	278	284	291	297	303	309	315	322	328	334
67	121	127	134	140	146	153	159	166	172	178	185	191	198	204	211	217	223	230	236	242	249	255	261	268	274	280	287	293	299	306	312	319	325	331	338	344
68	125	131	138	144	151	158	164	171	177	184	190	197	203	210	216	223	230	236	243	249	256	262	269	276	282	289	295	302	308	315	322	328	335	341	348	354
69	128	135	142	149	155	162	169	176	182	189	196	203	209	216	223	230	236	243	250	257	263	270	277	284	291	297	304	311	318	324	331	338	345	351	358	365
70	132	139	146	153	160	167	174	181	188	195	202	209	216	222	229	236	243	250	257	264	271	278	285	292	299	306	313	320	327	334	341	348	355	362	369	376
71	136	143	150	157	165	172	179	186	193	200	208	215	222	229	236	243	250	257	265	272	279	286	293	301	308	315	322	329	336	343	351	358	365	372	379	386
72	140	147	154	162	169	177	184	191	199	206	213	221	228	235	242	250	258	265	272	279	287	294	302	309	316	324	331	338	346	353	361	368	375	383	390	397
73	144	151	159	166	174	182	189	197	204	212	219	227	235	242	250	257	265	272	280	288	295	302	310	318	325	333	340	348	355	363	371	378	386	393	401	408
74	148	155	163	171	179	186	194	202	210	218	225	233	241	249	256	264	272	280	287	295	303	311	319	326	334	342	350	358	365	373	381	389	396	404	412	420
75	152	160	168	176	184	192	200	208	216	224	232	240	248	256	264	272	279	287	295	303	311	319	327	335	343	351	359	367	375	383	391	399	407	415	423	431
76	156	164	172	180	189	197	205	213	221	230	238	246	254	263	271	279	287	295	304	312	320	328	336	344	353	361	369	377	385	394	402	410	418	426	435	443

Source: Adapted from Clinical Guidelines on the Identification, Evaluation, and Treatment of Overweight and Obesity in Adults: The Evidence Report.

What Your BMI Means

Classifications	BMI
▶ Underweight	less than 18.5
▶ Normal weight	18.5–24.9
▶ Overweight	25.0–29.9
▶ Mild obesity	30.0–34.9
▶ Moderate obesity	35.0–39.9
▶ Extreme obesity	40.0 or greater

Take a look at the BMI classifications above and fill in the blanks: "I'm _____ because my BMI is _____." For example: "I'm moderately obese because my BMI is 37."

What's a Healthy Weight?

"Healthy" or "desirable" body weight: what exactly do these terms mean? You're at a healthy or desirable weight if you:

▶ meet the standards of a weight guideline such as *Dietary Guidelines for Healthy Americans,* or the Body Mass Index chart

▶ have the kind of body fat distribution that lowers your risk of disease or death, which means that your body shape is more like a pear than an apple

▶ are at a weight that doesn't cause you to develop an unhealthy medical condition

▶ have a BMI of less than 25

Here are some examples of healthy weights:

▶ 5'10" man, 165 lbs.
▶ 5'5" woman, 130 lbs.
▶ 5'6" adolescent boy, 140 lbs.
▶ 5'1" teenage girl, 115 lbs.

Overweight (BMI 25–29.9): To be considered overweight, you must weigh no more than 10 percent above the desirable weight for your height. Research shows that if your BMI is greater than 28, you're at much greater risk for stroke, heart disease, and type 2 diabetes.

Here are some examples of overweight:

- 5'10" man, 190 lbs.
- 5'5" woman, 160 lbs.
- 5'6" adolescent boy, 175 lbs.
- 5'1" teenage girl, 140 lbs.

Obese (BMI = 30 or greater): You are considered obese if your body weight is greater than 10 percent above the desirable weight for your height. There are three classes or degrees of obesity:

Class 1 (mild)	BMI = 30–34.9
Class 2 (moderate)	BMI = 35–39.9
Class 3 (extreme)	BMI = 40 or higher

Here are some examples of obese weights:

- 5'10" man, 220 lbs. (mild); 250 lbs. (moderate); 300 lbs. (severe)
- 5'5" woman, 190 lbs. (mild); 220 lbs. (moderate); 260 lbs. (severe)
- 5'6" adolescent boy, 190 lbs. (mild); 230 lbs. (moderate); 250 lbs. (severe)
- 5'1" teenage girl, 160 lbs. (mild); 190 lbs. (moderate); 220 lbs. (severe)

Health professionals often use a person's BMI to help them determine if that person's weight is a risk factor for poor health. Most of the time it serves as a reliable indicator; there are a few exceptions, though: some muscular athletes, pregnant women, and adolescents may, for reasons of extraordinary muscle and/or skeletal growth, as well as temporary maternal and fetal growth, have higher than desirable BMIs and yet not be unhealthy. Just to be sure, there's another body measurement that you can take right in your own home: It's your waist circumference.

Waist Circumference

In addition to BMI, waist circumference (the distance around your waist) is important, because research shows that extra abdominal fat is a serious risk factor for such health concerns as type 2 diabetes, high blood pressure, heart disease, and elevated cholesterol. The following waist measurements (once again, excluding pregnant women) indicate excess abdominal fat, which would put you at greater disease risk:

Men   40 inches or more
Women   35 inches or more

(Read more about body shapes on pages 93–94.)

Connection: Overworked, Overstressed, Overeating

It's hard to escape from the ever-present, widespread influences of super-sized, cheap, easy-to-grab, high-calorie foods that have infiltrated our meals at home and away from home. Our quick-paced days, with too much to do and too little time to do it in, encourages what has become a mindless way of eating. Meals are considered a low-priority chore or time constraint, or possibly a much-needed escape from a stressful day.

Our obesity statistics are soaring because we eat too much, move too little, and deal with sky-high levels of daily stress. Believe it or not, there was a time when, as Americans, life wasn't so hectic, when meals and mealtimes were actually given their importance throughout the day, three times a day. To illustrate this point, I've compared the typical schedules of Rose, a stay-at-home mom from the 1950s, and Mary, the new-millennium supermom. I think you'll agree: what a difference just fifty years can make!

Rose's Story

Rose was a happily married homemaker. She lived in a two-family house in an urban neighborhood, where her parents lived on the ground floor and she and her family above them. Her husband worked for a large furniture store in a big city. They had two teenage children; the son traveled forty-five minutes by train to his high school and the daughter walked to the local high school. Most stores were within walking distance. Rose had no major health problems, although some longstanding childhood illnesses had left her with mild anemia and some visual disability. In general, though, she lived the lifestyle of a strong, healthy forty-three-year-old woman. She was 5'1" tall and weighed 118 pounds, which comes out to a BMI of 22, a healthy weight. Here's what one of Rose's typical days looked like:

Morning

6:30: Woke up, prepared breakfast and lunches for the family

Breakfast: Orange juice, buttered toast, poached egg, cup coffee or glass whole milk

7:30–9:00: Sent family off to work or school; washed, dried, and put away breakfast dishes; swept kitchen floor; made beds; tidied up bathroom; put load of dirty laundry in washing machine (in the basement); got dressed in street clothes for daily marketing

9:00–11:00: Walked to the grocer, the butcher, and the bakery

11:00–11:15: Walked home, either carrying brown paper bundles or wheeling a pushcart depending on the number of items purchased

11:15–11:45: Delivered groceries to her mother and put away all bought items, went down to basement, unloaded washed laundry into basket, and hung clothes on outdoor laundry line

11:45–12:15: Prepared and ate lunch

Lunch: Ham and cheese sandwich on white bread with mustard, lettuce, and tomato, piece of fruit, water

Afternoon

12:15–12:30: Cleaned up after lunch and washed, dried, and put away dishes

12:30–1:30: Took a nap

1:30–3:00: Began prep work for dinner meal: Made salad; started homemade vegetable soup; cleaned whole chicken and prepared it for oven roasting; cut up roasting vegetables. Picked up dried laundry

3:00–3:15: Made snack for daughter arriving home from school, sprinkled water on laundry to be ironed

3:15–4:45: Put chicken roaster and vegetables in oven, ironed

4:45–5:00: Removed ironing board from kitchen, set dinner table, made final preparations for evening meal

Evening

5:15–5:30: Husband and son returned home, everyone washed up for dinner

5:30–6:15: Family ate dinner together

Dinner: Homemade vegetable barley soup, oven-roasted chicken, roasted potatoes and carrots, lettuce and tomato salad, homemade vinaigrette dressing, piece of fruit, water

6:15–6:45: Cleaned up, washed, dried, and put away dishes, folded and put away tablecloth and cloth napkins, swept floor

6:45–7:00: Made and served after-dinner dessert

Snack: Cup of coffee and coffee cake

7:00–9:00: Watched TV or read; mended if necessary

9:00–9:15: Washed up and went to bed

Keep in mind that in 1950, Rose had to do without these handy time- and energy-savers:

- Steam iron
- Remote control for the TV

- Clothes dryer
- Permanent press (no-iron) clothing
- One-stop megamarkets
- Food processor
- Convenience or prepared foods
- Microwave oven
- Dishwasher
- TV in the kitchen
- Takeout rotisserie chicken
- Precut packaged vegetables
- Prewashed bagged salads

So on this, one of Rose's typical days, she exercised (only she called it housekeeping, food shopping, doing the laundry, and ironing) for about six hours! That exercise included walking for at least thirty minutes and climbing at least two sets of stairs five times each. She ate three meals a day, which added up to about 1,600 calories, 38 percent fat (65 grams), and 20 grams of fiber. She got nine hours of sleep each night, and took a one-hour afternoon nap. Rose was happy with her life, contented with what she had, and wasn't looking for more than she needed.

Postscript: Rose was a real person who lived a healthy life until she died of natural causes at the age of ninety-three.

Mary's Story

Mary is a forty-something new-millennium supermom. She works as a full-time school administrator, is the mother of three children, ages ten to eighteen years old, and close to earning her master's degree in education. Her husband, a first responder, works shifts and rotates different work schedules every month. Mary has had high blood pressure for several years; she also recently found out that she has high cholesterol and triglycerides. Mary has also struggled with her weight for several years. She's 5'1" and weighs 145 pounds. (Her BMI is 27, which classifies her as overweight.)

Morning

5:45–6:40: Gets up, puts in load of laundry, walks with a friend around the neighborhood for about 40 minutes

6:40–8:10: Empties dishwasher, makes lunch for three kids, makes bed, gets ready for work, prepares breakfast for kids, eats breakfast herself, does whatever household chores time will allow (empty garbage, tidy up family room, or clip food coupons)

Breakfast: Two slices toast, 1 tbs. reduced fat peanut butter, 4-oz. glass orange juice, peach

8:10–8:45: Drives youngest child to school, puts first load of laundry into dryer, starts second load, makes lunch to bring to work

8:45–9:00: Carpools with co-worker

9:00–12:30: Observes class at one preschool

Afternoon

12:30–1:15: Lunch break

Lunch: Lettuce, ½ can water-packed tuna, 1 tbs. light dressing, orange, water

1:15–3:00: Writes observational report from the morning's class

3:00-3:20: Drops off co-worker (if it is her turn to drive), returns home

3:20–4:00: Eats snack with daughter and helps her with her homework

Snack: Six low-fat cookies

4:00–5:00: Prepares dinner

Evening

5:00–6:00: Serves and eats dinner with whichever family members are home

Dinner: Two slices grilled chicken breast, large helping steamed broccoli with spray butter, large plain baked potato, water

6:00–8:30: Meets with graduate school study group three nights a week; grocery-shops two nights a week; works on graduate studies or school projects if at home

8:30–9:30: Eats a snack, calls elderly parent or friend (if she's not too tired)

Snack: Small cup of fat-free chocolate pudding

9:30–10:30: Puts the ten-year-old to bed, folds laundry, prepares clothes and books for next day

10:30: Goes to bed (husband may or may not be at home)

As you can see, Mary has put in a long, exhausting, stressful day by anyone's standards. She couldn't possibly have squeezed in any more activities—she had no time or energy left! After just seven hours of sleep, she forces herself to get up for that morning walk. Here's what she says about that exercise time: "I make myself do it because I have to get my weight, blood pressure, and cholesterol down and I know exercise will help. But do you know what? The whole time I'm walking I'm either thinking to myself of all I have to do as soon as I get back home or, even worse, I'm complaining to my friend!"

Mary takes in about 1,300 calories, 21 percent fat (30 grams) and 17 grams of fiber, and probably burned about 220 calories on her walk. She admits that before her most recent doctor visit, she wasn't watching her diet: "It's so much easier to order takeout or bring the kids to McDonald's. I don't have the time or the energy to cook." She knows that she used food for comfort, so calories really didn't matter. High-fat, super-sized meals and snacks were the order of the day. But now she's proud of herself that she's walking and improving her diet.

Mary looks ahead to an easier daily pace. She admits, though, that taking it easy isn't in her immediate future: Her youngest child will be at home for several more years, her husband's erratic work schedule won't improve until he retires, and that's still many years away. She's concerned about her health; she realizes that the stress in her life impacts negatively on her health. She'd like to slow down and smell the roses—if only she could find the magic to make it happen.

As crazy as Mary's life seems, she's caught up in much the same vicious cycle as many of us. Her daily doings show how today's lifestyle (and all the "conveniences" of it) can lead us down a slippery slope toward overweight and obesity. Here's how:

▶ Most of us eat too many calories, sometimes for comfort or convenience, especially empty and high-fat calories. After all, it's easy to find cheap junk food just about anywhere, at any time, twenty-four hours a day, seven days a week. Worse yet, it's served in huge portions!

▶ Some of us go from eating too much to eating way too little, which also doesn't help us lose weight.

▶ We tend not to seize the opportunities embedded in our day to burn off some of the extra calories we've eaten.

▶ We're under way too much stress. It drains our energy and makes us feel tired, depressed, and sick.

The outlook may seem pretty bleak, but here's the positive spin: There's no magic involved, but if you're willing to think out of the *dieting* box, you could finally succeed at losing weight and keeping it off for the long haul by focusing on making small, consistent changes rather than fast-forwarding to the end result. *Aim for progress, not perfection.*

The 10% Solution

When "diet" describes a way of eating, it can have a positive meaning, as in "a high-fiber *diet*" or "a balanced *diet.*" But "diet," as in diet -*ing*, isn't such a positive word. Why is that, if excess weight is such a health concern for so many of us? Shouldn't we "diet"? No, because those kinds of "diets" don't work. You know that from your own past experience.

To lose weight and keep it off, you need to change your everyday habits. When you make gradual and reasonable changes, they become part of your lifestyle and don't feel like changes anymore. You won't feel deprived as new habits take hold because you won't feel as if you're sacrificing anything. It just becomes the way you eat.

Losing just 10 percent of your current body weight—*no matter how overweight you are*—will reduce your risk factors for diabetes, heart disease, and some forms of cancer. Let's call it the "10% Solution." Losing just the first two digits of your total weight will give you more energy and a new start on a longer, healthier life. I list some examples of a 10 percent weight loss below.

▶ **Person 1:** 5'1" tall and weighs **145** lbs. 10% = losing **14½** lbs.
▶ **Person 2:** 5'5" tall and weighs **200** lbs. 10% = losing **20** lbs.
▶ **Person 3:** 5'8" and weighs **280** lbs. 10% = losing **28** lbs.
▶ **Person 4:** 6' tall and weighs **310** lbs. 10% = losing **31** lbs.

These examples prove that you don't have to lose all your extra weight to feel better and improve your health. *Aim for progess, not perfection.*

> *Did You Know . . .* Scientists estimate that a lean adult body contains approximately *30 billion* fat calls; an adult obese body may have as many as *120 billion* fat cells!

A True Story (Male Version)

Chris, a middle-aged man, is 5'9" tall and weighs 224 pounds (his BMI is 33, making him mildly obese). He takes medications for high blood pressure and high cholesterol; he also has type 2 diabetes but isn't on any medication yet. At a recent checkup, his doctor discovered that Chris's blood pressure was elevated and a fingerstick blood test revealed a high glucose reading. He talked to his doctor about what he should do: They agreed that Chris should lose some weight. The doctor suggested that Chris set up an appointment with me; he agreed, without enthusiasm.

Chris didn't want to keep his nutrition counseling appointment; after all, he thought he already knew what I would say to him: "I know what she is going to tell me. I have to eat smaller portions, not eat out, not have any ice cream, and, and, and . . ." but Chris did keep his appointment. And this is what I said to him:

"You weigh 224 pounds today. Will you consider losing just 10 percent of your present weight—that's 22 pounds—over the next six months? That's actually less than a pound a week. Once you've lost the 22 pounds, I'll teach you how to maintain that loss for another six months, which means that one year from now you'll weigh 200 pounds. When was the last time you weighed so little? And if you take six months to lose 22 pounds, then take another six months to maintain that loss, chances are very good that you'll stay at 200 pounds forever. That is, unless you decide to lose another 10 percent!"

I didn't tell Chris to lose 60 pounds but instead suggested that he lose just 22, or 10 percent of his current body weight. Chris returned home feeling for the first time in his life that he really *could* lose those 22 pounds. He'd never felt so good about losing weight before. Ah-ha! *That* was the difference! After I outlined a meal plan for him and Chris realized that he had to work on just a few changes ("Work at your own pace. *Aim for progress, not perfection.*"), he didn't feel overwhelmed and definitely didn't feel like he was "dieting."

After living with the 10% Solution/"I'm not dieting" attitude for nine weeks, Chris had lost seven pounds and was well on his way to achieving his own 10% Solution. Besides losing weight, Chris was also reducing his risk of developing heart disease as well as further diabetes complications. Chris knows that he still has a weight problem, and that he'll still be overweight even after he loses those 22 pounds. But he also knows he's improving his health with every pound he loses. In fact, he now says to himself, "I can do this!" His small but consistent *changes* are becoming *habits* and those *habits* are developing into a *lifestyle*—one that just happens to encourage weight loss and good health.

How the 10% Solution Can Be Sabotaged

So, your goal is to lose weight to improve your health, not to look good for a wedding or a reunion or so you can look better in your bathing suit on vacation. You decide to try to lose just 10 percent of your current weight over a relatively long period of time—twelve months, to be exact. What's the easiest way to make this approach work?

There's no way around it: To lose weight, the number of calories *coming in* has to be less than the number of calories *going out*. You can do this in three different ways:

1. You can cut back on the calories you eat (fewer calories *in*).
2. You can increase your amount of exercise (more calories *out)*.
3. You can reduce the number of calories you're eating and exercise more (fewer calories *in* plus more calories *out*).

The problem is, if you go overboard and cut your calories too much and/or increase your exercise too much, before long you'll start feeling hungry and weak. You might get dizzy or shaky or develop headaches. To make matters worse, you might also notice that you aren't even losing weight. What's happening?

Our bodies learned ages and ages ago, when our ancestors faced famines, to store as much energy as they possibly could. As I explained in chapter 1, this is exactly what your body does with all excess calories; it turns them into body fat and that body fat becomes an energy reserve. Your body doesn't want to use its stored energy; in fact, it just wants to keep accumulating more and more.

When the number of calories that you're taking *in* is much less than the calories you're putting *out*, alarms go off inside your body, forcing it to preserve its stored fat. Keep in mind that your body still has to come up daily with the energy it needs for all its necessary functions and activities. Since you aren't getting enough calories, you have to dig into your energy reserves to meet your energy needs. *But your body doesn't want to resort to this.* So, first it sends out some warnings: You may get a headache or feel faint. These indicators are your body's way of saying "Feed me. Give me the calories I need to keep enough energy pumping into those working cells without using the reserves."

If the warnings go unheeded, your body can still do something to prevent major energy losses from its fat stores. And here comes the bad news: It can simply slow down the rate at which it uses energy—the energy it needs to keep your heart pumping and continue performing all the other tasks it has to do to keep you alive. (The rate that your body uses energy for all its functions is called the *basal metabolic rate.*) Your body is only doing what it has learned to do throughout evolution: conserve energy.

Now, back to you, the dieter: What's happened? With all good intentions, you go on your "diet," which means that you're drastically cutting calories and maybe even exercising as much as you can. Yes, you feel horrible after a few days, but because you're determined to lose weight *this time,* you keep at it. You watch the scale and, after going down a pound or two or three, the needle stops moving. Wanting more spectacular results, you get frustrated and give up the "diet." You decide that you lack willpower, it's just too hard to lose weight, or there's something metabolically wrong with you, or all of the above. There's nothing wrong with you, but a lot wrong with your approach to losing weight. What do you need to be convinced that *diets don't work?*

QUOTE OF THE DAY:
*"I have not failed.
I've just found 10,000 ways that won't work."*
—Thomas Edison

Tricklers and the 10% Solution

To succced at losing weight, your body must work with you, not against you, during your deliberate energy shortage. Your brain interprets how much energy it has to work with by the level of glucose in your blood. If enough calories aren't coming *in,* then the new supply of energy won't be enough. And as the glucose in your blood gets used up, your glucose level drops, and your brain interprets this drop as "hunger." In other words, your brain wants you to eat more food so that it can receive a new supply of energy.

Your brain also registers hunger when there is a sharp rise in blood glucose followed by a rapid drop. This is exactly what happens after eating quickly digested carbs that require significant insulin activity, and it reacts the same way it does when there is a calorie shortage, even though this isn't the case. A large amount of insulin responds to the large amount of glucose entering your blood. Unfortunately, you don't necessarily burn the glucose pulled out of your blood; if there's too much, you store it as fat. But because your blood-glucose level has been lowered, your brain wants you to eat more food so that it can renew its energy supply.

Question: What causes this continual hunger cycle?
Answer: The roller-coaster effect of high blood-glucose levels followed by high insulin levels in the blood resulting in drastically lowered levels of glucose in the blood.

Question: Is this blood-glucose roller-coaster good or bad?
Answer: It's bad if you're trying to lose weight, because now your body (thanks to your brain's alertness) goes into "preservation mode" to store as much energy as it can rather than burn as much energy as it can.

Question: Why does your body want to store energy?
Answer: Because it's afraid you'll starve: It's been preprogrammed to store as much glucose as it can when blood levels are low, regardless of *why* they're low.

Question: Can you prevent this from happening?
Answer: Yes!

We gain weight because we are eating too much of everything. But if we cut back our portions we may feel hungry. Enter the tricklers, those slowly digested carbs that your body turns into glucose in a slow, steady way. Here is how trickler carbs arrest hunger. By supplying a steady stream of glucose to the blood, which then sends this steady glucose supply to the working cells that are looking for it, your brain isn't registering "hunger" because your blood-glucose levels never dip low (unless four or five hours have passed since you ate and it's time to eat again). Also, tricklers tend to physically stay in the gut longer, promoting a sense of fullness.

To succeed at losing weight, you should not feel hungry. Tricklers keep you from feeling hungry.

In order to lose weight and keep it off, you don't want to feel those energy highs and the inevitable lows; instead, you need to have a consistent, steady supply of glucose to meet your endless energy needs. Tricklers are the best carb choices for keeping up a steady energy supply—even over a period of several hours. And when you keep getting the energy you need, those highs and lows become a thing of the past: You don't feel headachy or light-headed, and you have plenty of energy to make it through the day and night. When your body gets what it needs from the food you eat, it's in harmony and gives you a great feeling of well being. Tricklers give you a sense of control. You can say to yourself, "Hey! I can do this!"

To succeed at losing weight, you must feel good. Tricklers allow you to feel in control and enjoy a sense of well being.

You gradually have to use some of your fat stores in order to lose weight. By causing a slower, smaller, and steadier rise in blood-glucose levels, tricklers keep your body from pumping a surge of insulin into your bloodstream. The result? Your cells will get just the right amount of sugar *as they need it*—no less and no more. If too much glucose dumps into your blood (and, as a result, too much insulin as well), what happens to it if you don't need it right then? Insulin delivers it to the liver, where it's converted into fat. This explains how gushers can add to fat stores, and why tricklers don't.

To succeed at losing weight, you must gradually use some of your stored fat. Tricklers help your body use this stored fat.

No food is bad. But the case remains strong: Carbohydrates are your body's fuel of choice. As you already know, in a healthy, balanced diet, the majority of your calories should come from carbohydrates. That's why carbohydrates are the single most influential nutrient you can eat; they affect your day-to-day living as well as your general health. To keep your weight under control, then, you need to look at the types of carbs you're eating. And tricklers, the low-GI carbohydrates, are the best types of carbs to help you lose weight and keep it off. You can take a peek at some low-GI meals and snacks by turning to pages 136–142.

A True Story (Female Version)

Amy, a thirty-something administrative assistant, came to see me about her diabetes. With a strong family history of the disease on both maternal and paternal sides, she was worried how diabetes might play out in her body. She was not on medication for it as yet, but her doctor was not optimistic about the future unless things changed. Amy hoped there would be a way to control the disease naturally. Not a "pills person," she was taking blood pressure medication and "not happy about it." She also admitted that she was very concerned about her weight. She had been contemplating gastric bypass surgery.

Amy stood 5'7" tall and weighed 320 pounds. Her BMI measured 50, indicating extreme obesity. Determined to improve her health, Amy started to walk outside her office building on her lunch hour. She made valiant efforts every day to cut back on calories, but she'd get so hungry that she'd grab some chocolate candies from her boss's desk or snack on cake or doughnuts. By the time she came to see me, Amy had become a faithful visitor to her company's fitness center, spending 45 minutes of her lunch hour every day doing both cardiac and resistance training workouts. Her pumped-up exercise routine was working: she had lost 36 pounds. But she was always hungry and knew that she needed to straighten out her diet.

Constructing a typical day's 24-hour food and drink diary was difficult for Amy. She never considered portions: she either ate what was served to her or as much food as she felt like having. She ate through her emotions, especially when she was sad or angry or tired. Yet, she weighed herself everyday without fail, which only strengthened the depression she felt about her weight.

From what I could tell, Amy was not a fussy eater, she enjoyed her fruits and vegetables, and her meals were balanced until dinner. The evening meal tended to be large portions of fat-laden foods. I listened attentively as she rattled off the carbohydrate foods she ate most frequently. As expected, several gushers were showing up regularly (and in large amounts) on her plate: pineapple, watermelon, fruit juices, doughnuts, bagels, and Italian bread.

Here was my chance to kill two birds with one stone for Amy. I explained to her how she could regulate her blood-glucose levels by incorporating and regulating the amounts of whole grains, fruits, vegetables, and low-fat dairy foods into her day, exchanging her usual quickly digested carbs for the more slowly digested ones. I explained how tricklers would prevent blood glucose spikes, help her feel satisfied, calm and "in control," and encourage her body to burn fat rather than store it. In other words, I clarified that by improving her diet, both her diabetes and weight concerns would be addressed simultaneously.

I won't say that Amy jumped for joy and was full of excitement; sometimes I see this in patients who are afraid to believe that "*this time*" may be the right time to lose weight effectively. But together we strategized a game plan. The changes were clear-cut: she would start to decrease or eliminate the high-GI fruits and replace them with trickler fruits; breads would be whole grain; the evening meal would consist of smaller starch and protein portions, and she promised to cover half of her plate with vegetables. We agreed that this might be all that she needed to do, especially since she already had a well-established commitment to exercise and had healthy water-drinking habits.

In fact, as things turned out, that *was* all Amy needed! In a little over one year, she has lost 118 pounds! Her most recent blood work results showed a 31 percent jump in her HDL (good cholesterol), a 74 percent drop in triglycerides and a 26 percent drop in mean glucose levels. She is on no medication, works out six days a week ("I just love my spinning classes!"), has no more joint pains, and feels great.

So great that Amy is thinking of becoming a spinning class instructor—"just part-time."

Are You Motivated to Lose Weight?

Did you know that the weakest motivator for shedding pounds is just *wanting* to? It's almost as if a little voice says, "Who are you trying to kid? Sure you'll be 'good' for a week or two, but come on; you know it's not going to work. Why should it? You've never kept lost weight off before!" After listening to that internal voice, who wouldn't feel defeated from the very start? On the other hand, you're more strongly motivated to lose weight if you want to . . .

Keep your good health. "Diabetes runs in my family. If I keep my weight down, I'll improve my odds of not getting it myself."

Improve your health. "My doctor told me that if I could lose some weight, my blood pressure would improve and I might not need to take any medication."

Boost your energy level. "If only I weren't so tired, maybe I could make dinner tonight and even go for a bike ride with the kids after school. But I'm exhausted. These extra 50 pounds I carry around all day long wear me out. I know that if I could lose some weight, I'd have more energy and feel younger too."

The Successful-Loser Profile

In 1993 the National Weight Control Registry began to track people eighteen years and older who had lost at least 30 pounds and successfully kept it off for a minimum of one year. To date, the registry has listed about 3,000 people. The average registrant has lost approximately 67 pounds and has successfully maintained that loss for about six years. Here's how these successful losers did it:

Eighty-nine percent watched their fat intake, controlled portion sizes, and burned an average of 400 calories a day, usually by walking.

To learn more about the National Weight Control Registry, call 1-800-606-NWCR (6927) or visit: www.uchsc.edu/nutrition/ WyattJortberg/nwcr.htm.

A Word About Low-Carb Diets

There are indications that the low-carb diet trend is finally starting to wind down. After all I've explained about carbohydrates being the body's fuel of choice, I hope you will agree with me that this can only be a good thing for all bodies. Our bodies have been built to run on a specific kind of fuel: glucose. And the body has chosen carbohydrates, not proteins or fats, as its preferred fuel source. No best-selling diet book will change this fact! By returning carbs back into the system, the body has a fighting chance to have the energy it needs to support and maintain itself and burn calories at a metabolically healthy rate.

Since most of the calories we use throughout the day are spent on metabolic activity (heart, lung, blood, digestive organs etc.), we don't want to decrease this activity in any way, especially when trying to lose weight. Because, in the end, there is only one equation for weight loss:

*Calories **in** must be **less than** calories **out**.*

It is the overwhelming consensus of the research community that diets that are low or moderate in fats and high in carbohydrates tend to be lower in calories.

And the slowly digested carbs will never fail your weight loss attempts: they provide you with consistent energy *even though you are in an energy deficit*, they keep your belly feeling full, and they assist your cells in burning fat rather than storing it. You're not dragging, you're not hungry or in a bad mood, and you're chipping away at the excess fat! What more could you ask for in a permanent plan to lose weight?

Since lifestyle changes, not diets, promote lasting weight loss, which lifestyle do you prefer: no pasta, potatoes, bread, fruit or ice cream *forever*, or small portions of your preferred carbs throughout your day, *every day*? I know my answer!

A postscript to those die-hard, carb-counters out there: Don't be fooled by the "net carb," "net impact carb," "useable carb," even "low-carb" marketing gimmick. These are not terms that have been defined by the FDA; they have been invented by the companies selling these products! So no one is regulating their use, at least, not yet. But, as long as you're looking at nutrition information labels on your favorite low-carb, maybe no-carb bread, cereal, cookie, or ice cream, ask yourself what was substituted when the carbs were taken out. You're staring at the answer: fat and or protein, and very often, many more calories!

Looking for the secret formula for maintaining lost weight?

DO exercise

DO eat a balanced diet focusing on low-GI carbs

DON'T forget what being "fat" felt like

THE BOTTOM LINE

➤ The body's fuel of choice is carbohydrates.

➤ The body is not programmed to extract immediate energy from proteins or fats.

➤ Losing just 10 percent of your extra weight will help you feel better and improve your health.

➤ Tricklers are the best types of carbs in a balanced diet to help you lose weight and keep it off, by keeping your energy up and excessive calories down.

➤ The most successful dieters have made a permanent commitment to exercise and portion control.

6

CONTROL YOUR BLOOD SUGAR THE GOOD-CARB WAY

Do you have diabetes? Eighteen million Americans do, even though more than 5 million of them don't know it yet. *Every day*, more than 3,500 people across the United States are diagnosed with diabetes. In the last decade alone, the incidence of type 2 diabetes, the most prevalent form of diabetes, shot up 40 percent! Among the thirty-something crowd, there's been an estimated 70 percent increase! And more than 200,000 young Americans under the age of twenty have been diagnosed with diabetes, including both types 1 and 2.

With such staggering statistics, it is understandable that this disease has accelerated to the sixth leading cause of death, with an annual cost of $132 billion and taking more American lives in one year than the entire nine-year Vietnam War conflict.

What Is Diabetes?

Diabetes is a chronic disease that results from a lack of, or ineffective use of, insulin. Insulin, to review, escorts glucose, protein-building molecules, and fat-storing molecules (from carbohydrate, protein, and fat digestion, respectively) into cells to meet your ongoing energy and health maintenance needs.

Here's an easier way to describe the disease: If you have diabetes, your body has difficulty removing glucose from your bloodstream and getting it into your cells so they can use it for energy. This happens because your body either doesn't produce enough insulin or uses it ineffectively or both. Without the right supply of insulin, blood levels of glucose will rise. This elevated blood-glucose level is called *hyperglycemia*.

hyper = high
glyc = sugar
emia = blood

So as food enters your body and your gut digests it, glucose, amino acids, and fatty acids dump into your bloodstream. If your insulin supply can't meet the glucose demand or if your body cells are resisting insulin's action, your glucose levels begin to rise. If these levels go high enough and stay that way for an extended period of time, the classic symptoms of high blood glucose, or *hyperglycemia,* show up.

Types of Diabetes

Diabetes can be classified into three different types, all of which are different diseases. People with any form of diabetes may experience some of the same symptoms, however, and share common risk factors for prolonged complications.

Type 1 Diabetes

Type 1 diabetes used to be called insulin-dependent diabetes, or juvenile-onset diabetes. This form of the disease usually occurs before age thirty but can happen at any age. The classic symptoms of increased hunger and thirst, frequent urination, fatigue, and weight loss appear suddenly. Specialized cells in your pancreas have stopped producing insulin, so you must take daily insulin injections to survive. Five to 10 percent of people with diabetes have type 1.

Type 2 Diabetes

Type 2 diabetes is referred to as non-insulin-dependent diabetes, or adult-onset diabetes. This type of diabetes usually occurs after age thirty but can also affect children and adolescents (a trend that's becoming more widespread as overweight and obesity rates for children and adolescents continue to rise). Ninety to 95 percent of people who have diabetes have type 2. The disease is more common in certain ethnic groups such as Africans, Latinos, Native Americans, and Pacific Islanders. Overweight and obese people are at higher risk of developing type 2 diabetes.

If you have this form of the disease, you may experience blurred vision, numbness, tingling in the hands and feet, slow wound healing, recurring yeast infections, or itchy skin. Sometimes you can control type 2 diabetes by making some lifestyle changes to your eating and exercise habits. Some people may also need medication, even insulin, to control the disease.

Gestational Diabetes

Gestational diabetes results from carbohydrate intolerance due to insulin resistance during pregnancy. It usually occurs between the 24th and 28th weeks of pregnancy and occurs in 2 to 5 percent of all pregnancies in the United States. Women with gestational diabetes are considered at high risk, and since there may be no physical symptoms, a blood test is performed on all pregnant women. Although the disease disappears once the baby is born, approximately 40 percent of these women who were obese before pregnancy will develop type 2 diabetes within four years.

Prediabetes

It is estimated by the National Institute of Diabetes and Digestive and Kidney Diseases that 41 million middle-aged Americans (one in five) have prediabetes. People with this condition may show no symptoms, but a blood test will provide the diagnosis. If you have prediabetes, here's what your blood test results will show:

- fasting glucose test (110–125 mg/dl)
- oral glucose tolerance test (140–199 mg/dl)

Prediabetes is a hallmark characteristic of a condition known as the metabolic syndrome (see chapter 7). If left untreated, it will most likely develop into type 2 diabetes. There is good news, though, concerning this worrisome diagnosis. Studies from Harvard University have shown that by adopting a healthy lifestyle and losing excess weight, the risk of developing diabetes drops 55 percent.

It is important for physicians to realize that patients with cardiovascular disease may also have prediabetes. Proper diagnosis will lead to appropriate treatment. This gives the patient the best chance of avoiding future diabetes-related complications.

A Myth Dispelled

Question: If I eat too many sweets, will I get diabetes?
Answer: No.

Warning Signs of Diabetes

Type 1
➤ Extreme fatigue
➤ Unusual thirst
➤ Frequent urination
➤ Extreme hunger
➤ Unusual weight loss
➤ Irritability

Type 2
➤ Any type 1 symptoms
➤ Frequent infections
➤ Blurred vision
➤ Slow-to-heal cuts, bruises
➤ Tingling or numbness in hands or feet

Brain Teaser

Question: Which of the symptoms listed above do most people experience even before they're diagnosed with type 2 diabetes?
Answer: Tingling or numbness in hands or feet.

A Silent Killer

How can people have diabetes and not know it? Well, some people with type 2 diabetes may have no symptoms for a long time, maybe even years, or if they do, those symptoms are common enough to be explained away without much thought. Here are some of the disease's most common trademarks and how easy it is to ignore them:

Extreme fatigue. *How you might ignore the sign:* "Sure I'm tired. But I put in a long day. And I'm not getting any younger." *What is happening in your body:* Glucose isn't getting into your cells, yet they need to keep working anyway, so you end up feeling tired.

Unusual thirst. *How you might ignore the sign:* "I've always been a big drinker. And anyway, I thought water was good for you." *What is happening in your body:* Getting more water is your body's attempt to dilute the concentrated amount of sugar in your blood.

Frequent urination, especially at night. *How you might ignore the sign:* "Doesn't everybody have to get up at least a few times during the night?" *What is happening in your body:* If you drink a lot of liquids because you're thirsty, you'll need to get rid of that liquid, too.

Extreme appetite. *How you might ignore the sign:* "I must really be burning a lot of calories; I always seem to be hungry, even right after I've finished a meal." *What is happening in your body:* Because glucose isn't getting into your cells, your body thinks it needs more calories to get the energy it needs and knows that it can get more calories by signaling you to eat more.

Unexplained weight loss. *How you might ignore the sign:* "So what? I have to lose weight anyway." *What is happening in your body:* As blood-glucose levels keep rising higher and higher, your body desperately tries to get rid of some glucose, so it does the unthinkable: It excretes it! The calories you lose in your urine make you lose weight.

The Scope of the Problem

It may be easy to dismiss diabetes symptoms, but ignoring them doesn't make them go away. In fact, once you have diabetes, it *never* goes away.

In addition to the staggering number of diagnosed and undiagnosed diabetes cases, and the rapidly rising number of Americans with prediabetes "brewing" in their bodies, there is also a huge problem of diabetes among young people. In fact, increasingly more adolescents and even children as young as eight years of age are now being diagnosed with type 2 diabetes, which traditionally has been considered a disease of middle age. In the past five years alone, because of troubling overweight statistics, researchers have seen a tenfold increase in diabetes incidence in children. Type 2 diabetes in childhood, adolescence, or early adulthood is a particular concern because the earlier the disease takes hold, the longer the body has to potentially develop its complications.

The Diabetes Epidemic: Why Now?

You know the answer already: As a country, we eat too much and move around too little. In fact, it's no small wonder that Shape Up America!, a nonprofit organization that promotes healthy weight, coined the term "diabesity." The term stresses how important a trigger obesity is for the development of type 2 diabetes. And many of us also suffer from too much stress and fatigue, and chronic sleep deprivation.

But these problems are common, so why don't we all suffer from diabetes? Because only some people inherit the gene that makes the disease more likely to develop. For these people, the negative aspects of a fast-paced, computer-chipped, chocolate-chipped, potato-chipped, super-sized lifestyle may eventually get the better of them, and their bodies succumb to diabetes.

How Does Diabetes Start?

No one really knows what causes diabetes, which is why there's still no cure for it. Advances in medical science keep improving our understanding of diabetes, though, and we certainly know a lot more now than we did eighty years ago, when insulin was a new discovery. We know what to do to control the risk factors associated with diabetes and, perhaps more important, we're learning behavioral and medical strategies (for example, diet and combination drug therapy) to lessen our risk factors for *developing* the disease.

Question: What causes you to lose your ability to use glucose properly?

Answer: There are several possible causes of diabetes. Here are a few of them:

1. You could have inherited a gene that makes the disease more likely to develop.
2. You may have been exposed to an environmental trigger such as stress, toxins, or a virus, which could cause your body to destroy its own insulin-making cells in the pancreas (called an autoimmune reaction).
3. Your cells could become resistant to insulin.
4. Your pancreas could be secreting less insulin.
5. Your liver could be producing too much glucose.
6. Your diabetes could be caused by a combination of several of the factors listed above.

Who's at Risk for Diabetes?

You are at greater risk for developing type 1 diabetes if you have:

➤ A brother or sister with type 1

➤ At least one parent with type 1

You are at greater risk for developing type 2 diabetes if you:

➤ Have a family history of diabetes

➤ Are older than age forty-five

➤ Are overweight or obese, and are apple-shaped

➤ Are inactive

➤ Have high triglycerides

➤ Have low HDL (good) cholesterol

➤ Have had gestational diabetes or gave birth to a baby weighing nine or more pounds

➤ Are a member of certain racial and ethnic groups, such as an African American, Latino, Native American, Asian, and Pacific Islander

Why not . . . take the Diabetes Risk Test: http://diabetes.org/risk-test.jsp

Carbohydrates: Good Guys or Bad Guys?

It's a fact that your diet will impact your diabetes management. Hopefully this book is giving you some ideas for positive-impact strategies. If you're eating a healthy balanced diet, the majority of your calories are coming from carbohydrates. Your body loves to break down carbs into glucose; it's the easiest way your body knows to get energy without working too hard. For this reason, carbohydrates are your body's fuel of choice. This means that your body is willing to take every crumb or drop of any carbohydrate that you consume and break it down into glucose.

Thanks to extensive glycemic index research, we know that even though all carbs wind up in your blood as glucose, some types of carbs get there sooner than others. And if you have diabetes, a steep, rapid rise (or gush) in blood glucose can present a real problem: If your body has trouble moving the glucose into your cells and too much remains in your blood, it can lead to serious problems for your eyes, your kidneys, your peripheral nerves, and your heart.

So the bottom line is that, while no food is bad, the quickly digested carbs that I've been calling "gushers" will make blood-glucose control more difficult. That doesn't make them bad foods but rather less effective choices for blood-glucose control most of the time.

Did You Know . . . that blood-glucose levels fluctuate all the time? It's perfectly normal for the glucose level in the blood to rise 40 points after a meal.

Tricklers, the Superheroes

The more slowly glucose trickles into your blood, the easier it is for your body to manage this expected rise. If you've eaten slowly digested carbs, your body won't be overwhelmed with an onslaught of glucose molecules that need to move from your blood into your cells. And your body's insulin response can better handle the small, steady flow of glucose from these slowly digested carbs.

To summarize: With trickler carbs, glucose molecules enter your bloodstream gradually; insulin slowly escorts them from your blood into your cells. Slowly digested carbs make blood-glucose control easier. And not only do tricklers help to control blood-glucose levels, they also provide you with fiber, vitamins, minerals, and phytochemicals that contribute to the health of the rest of your body too. I think that qualifies these foods as nutritional superheroes.

Do Tricklers Work in Real Life?

Babs, seventy, mother of three and grandmother of six, has been married for forty-seven years. She works as a part-time book-keeper for the same small, family-owned sheet metal company where she has been employed for the past twenty-five years.

Babs is 5′4″; her weight had been steadily creeping up over the past several years to reach a record high of 229 pounds. (With a BMI of 39, she was moderately obese.) Because she carries her excess weight right around her middle, she is the perfect insulin-resistant "apple." (Studies show that excessive abdominal fat weakens insulin's ability to deliver glucose into the cells.) Twenty-three years ago, she was diagnosed with type 2 diabetes and started taking insulin three years later, after trying in vain to control her blood sugars with diet and pills. A biker and walker, Babs found herself becoming progressively more tired and wanting to do less and less physical activity. She injected herself with 25 units of insulin twice a day and saw blood-glucose readings ranging from 67 to 219, indicating poor control. She was also taking three medications to help control her high blood pressure.

Because Babs didn't know what she was doing wrong and didn't know how to make health improvements, she talked to her doctor and decided to get some nutritional counseling.

Babs's Diet: Before Carb Counseling

Breakfast: One-half grapefruit, 2 cups of regular coffee with half-and-half
Snack: Buttered roll, cup of regular coffee
Lunch: Small can tuna, 6 Triscuits, 12 oz. V-8 juice, 8 mini chocolate chip cookies
Snack: Orange
Dinner: Fried chicken breast, cup of rice with gravy, cup of tea
Snack: Three coconut macaroons

At first glance, Babs's diet doesn't seem too bad: two fruit servings, lean protein choices (tuna, chicken breast), and V-8, although high in sodium. When you add them up, Babs ate about 2,300 calories, and 45 percent of them were coming from fats. Her average daily diet pretty much kept her at her current weight, but since Babs was already moderately obese, she should lose weight to become healthier. And because she continued to feel too tired to exercise, the stage was set for Babs to keep gaining weight, which would worsen her insulin resistance. Increased insulin resistance would, in turn, continue to raise her blood-glucose levels, leaving her feeling hungry and tired, and continuing the vicious cycle.

How Could Babs Improve Her Diet?

The first thing Babs could do to help herself would be to start her day with a well-balanced breakfast, which would rev up her "motor" and start her burning as many calories as possible from the very beginning of the day. Then, by reducing her fat intake and introducing more tricklers into her diet (especially by eating whole-grain breads and crackers, and including vegetables and low-fat dairy products), Babs's blood-glucose levels would stabilize and she wouldn't feel so hungry. She would feel satisfied with fewer calories and would eat less. The result? Babs should start to lose weight and gradually become less insulin resistant. Both of these changes would improve her blood-sugar control as well as her quality of life.

Babs's Diet: After Carb Counseling

Breakfast: One-half cup old-fashioned oats cooked in a cup of 1% milk, ½ cup natural applesauce, regular coffee with fat-free half-and-half
Snack: Four Social Tea biscuits, decaf coffee
Lunch: Two oz. lean roast beef sandwich on 2 slices 100% stoneground whole wheat bread with lettuce, tomato, and mustard; a sandwich-sized bag of cut-up raw vegetables; water
Snack: Eight oz. light yogurt, ¾ cup honeydew and cantaloupe
Dinner: Three oz. grilled salmon, small grilled yam, 2 cups broccoli, small baked apple with cinnamon
Snack: Four oz. 1% milk, oatmeal cookie

It's hard to believe: All the food in Babs's "after" diet adds up to 600 *fewer* calories than her previous day's diet. The amounts of fruits and vegetables, dairy servings, and high-fiber, slowly digested tricklers increased as her fat and calorie intake greatly decreased. These foods amount to 1,700 calories, and 24 percent fat.

Babs: Down 42 Pounds and Feeling Great!

After just four months of dietary changes, Babs lost twenty pounds. It's now been nearly four years since she changed her dietary habits and she has lost 42 pounds! That terrific weight-loss success brought with it some wonderful health benefits: Babs went off *all insulin after just four months* of low-GI meal planning; she has not needed any insulin injections since then and her doctor has reduced her oral diabetes medication, too. Her blood-glucose levels have stabilized and now fall completely within the normal range. Another bonus: Because of her weight loss, Babs's blood pressure has returned to normal and her doctor has reduced those medications too.

So all of the health conditions that have caused Babs concern over the years have quickly improved: Her weight, blood-glucose levels, and blood pressure have all plummeted. The only thing that hasn't taken a nosedive is her spirits: "When I was too tired to do anything, I just didn't know who I was anymore. Now I feel really great—just like a teenager!"

Babs is one clear example that eating a healthful, balanced diet with low-GI foods works in real life!

THE BOTTOM LINE

➤ If your body doesn't produce enough insulin or uses it ineffectively, you will likely develop diabetes.

➤ There are three types of diabetes: type 1, type 2, and gestational.

➤ The prevalence of prediabetes, an insulin-resistant condition that results from excess weight and obesity, is currently on the rise.

➤ Quickly digested carbs, gushers, make blood-glucose control more difficult.

➤ Slowly digested carbs, tricklers, make blood-glucose control easier.

GOOD CARBS:
YOUR KEY TO A HEALTHIER HEART

Did you know that coronary heart disease (CHD) has been the #1 killer of American men and women every year since 1900 (except in 1918)? Today more than 2,500 people die of heart disease every day (one every 34 seconds), which added up to 700,000 deaths in 2001. High blood pressure, a major risk factor for heart disease, affects about 20 percent of the population.

But now did you also know that most Americans have their cholesterol checked by their doctors and that millions of people are taking medication that effectively lowers LDL ("bad") cholesterol? Research has proven that lowering LDL levels of cholesterol can reduce the risk for short-term heart disease by as much as 40 percent. But as the table below indicates, many of us need to decrease our numbers even further.

Patient Profile	LDL Goal*
Extremely high-risk	< 70 mg/dl
High-risk	< 100 mg/dl
Moderately high-risk	< 130 mg/dl
Low-risk	< 130 mg/dl

* These are the 2004 revised guidelines of the National Cholesterol Education Program Expert Panel on Detection, Evaluation, and Treatment of High Blood Cholesterol in Adults. They are based on a review of five major clinical trials of statin therapy for cholesterol management. While statins are a type of drug that can dramatically lower LDL cholesterol levels, the experts on this panel still emphasize an intensified use of nutrition, physical activity and weight control in the treatment of elevated cholesterol, something they call a "Therapeutic Lifestyle Changes" (or TLC) treatment plan.

So the message is: Heart disease kills but it doesn't have to kill *you*. That is, as long as you go for regular checkups, eat a healthful diet, make a commitment to regular exercise, and take prescribed medications, if recommended.

What Is Coronary Heart Disease?

Coronary heart disease is the most common form of heart disease. It is the number one killer of both men and women in the United States. This form of heart disease results from the narrowing of one or both of the coronary arteries that feed oxygen, and glucose to your heart. Over time, your arteries may become hard and stiff. Although physicians call this narrowing *atherosclerosis,* most of us know it as hardening of the arteries. People used to think that atherosclerosis was just a natural consequence of growing older, but the chronic buildup of plaque and the resulting hardened arteries and decreased, even blocked, blood flow to the heart is showing up even among young people in the prime of their lives! We know this because the incidence of heart attacks, high blood pressure, angina, and other related conditions is rising, even among young people.

What Narrows Arteries?

Arteries become narrow when there is a buildup of plaque, which are deposits made mostly of cholesterol, fats, and cells. If you have a lot of cholesterol in your blood, these deposits get bigger over time and narrow the arteries' passageway. That narrowing eventually reduces blood flow to your heart, which needs an uninterrupted supply of food and oxygen to function properly. Too much cholesterol blocks arteries and can cause heart pain (angina) or a heart attack.

What can cause an artery to become completely clogged? A lot of plaque buildup or a large blood clot. And blood clots are more likely to form in arteries with heavy plaque buildup. Any way you look at it, whether it is because of clogging or clotting, cholesterol is usually at least partly to blame.

Are You at Risk?

Several factors contribute to your heart disease risk, many of which you can control by eating well and getting more exercise. Two risk factors, though, your genes and your age, you can do nothing about.

It runs in the family. If heart disease affects other members of your family, you, too, may have inherited the same genetic tendency as some of your relatives. If your father or brother had premature heart disease (before age fifty-five) or your mother or sister had heart disease (before age sixty-five), there's a strong possibility that you have inherited this risk factor.

You're getting older. Once men reach age forty-five and women reach fifty-five, their age becomes a risk factor for heart disease. And no matter how many fountain-of-youth products you use, nothing can change your body's age.

> ✔ **Interested in estimating** your 10-year risk for developing coronary heart disease? Try this interactive Web site: http://hin.nhlbi.nih.gov/atpiii/calculator.asp

The Risk Factors You Can Control

You can improve your heart health by focusing on those risk factors you *can* control: cholesterol, blood pressure, elevated blood-glucose levels, weight, smoking, and stress (notice how many of these factors are diet-related). Here are nine strategies to work into your new, healthful lifestyle or your "Therapeutic Lifestyle Changes" treatment plan:

Heart-Health Strategy #1:
Lower Total and LDL (Bad) Cholesterol

If your total cholesterol is more than 200 mg/dl, and your LDL cholesterol is above 130 mg/dl, here is what to do to reduce both those numbers:

Limit amounts of high-fat animal products. Some fatty foods include spare ribs, sausage, hot dogs, burgers, bacon, salami, bologna, butter, whole-milk cheese, and whole-milk products.

Limit saturated fats. Sometimes we don't know that we're even eating saturated fats because they're hidden in prepared foods such as pastries, cookies, pies, gravies, and cream sauces. Eat these foods in moderation if at all.

Try replacing butter or regular stick margarines with plant stanols and sterols. These are plant-based natural substances that have been endorsed by the American Heart Association, among others, as effective aids in lowering cholesterol levels and reducing the risk of heart disease. Two to three grams daily of margarines like Benecol or Take Control are recommended.

Avoid trans fats. You can recognize trans fats if you read something such as "partially hydrogenated vegetable oil" on the food's ingredient list. Some foods that may contain trans fats include shortening, margarines, crackers, and cookies.

Cook the low-fat way. Bake, broil, grill, or steam your foods. For new ideas, buy some health magazines or visit these Web sites for some low-fat recipes to try:

> www.CookingLight.com
> www.intellihealth.com
> www.deliciousdecisions.org
> www.nhlbi.gov
> www.allrecipes.com
> www.mealsforyou.com

Eat more high-fiber foods. Some high-fiber superstars include vegetables, fruits, and whole grains.

Visit the user-friendly Web site created by the National Heart, Lung, and Blood Institute for more advice: www.nhlbi.nih.gov/chd/

> ***Did You Know. . .*** Foods derived from plants such as grains, cereals, fruits, and vegetables don't contain cholesterol. Only animals and foods made from animals contain cholesterol.

Heart-Health Strategy #2:
Increase HDL (Good) Cholesterol

Because HDL cholesterol protects against heart disease, the higher the number, the better. A level less than 40 mg/dl is low and is considered a major risk factor because it increases your risk for developing heart disease. If your levels are a bit on the low side, here's how you can pull them up:

Include monounsaturated and omega-3 fats in your daily diet. They help to protect your HDL levels. Keep in mind, though, that overdoing it won't give you extra protection, just extra calories. Good sources of monounsaturated fats include olive and canola oils, avocado, natural unsalted peanut butter, peanuts, and almonds. And good sources of omega-3 fats include wild or canned salmon, light tuna, sardines, flaxseed, and walnuts.

Get more exercise. Research shows that exercise can boost levels of this good cholesterol.

Stop smoking. Cigarette smoking, already a risk factor for heart disease, can also bring good cholesterol levels down. (It's never too late to kick the habit.)

The National Cholesterol Education Program Cholesterol Guidelines for Non-Diabetics

Total Cholesterol Number	Category
Less than 200 mg/dl*	Desirable
200–239 mg/dl	Borderline high
240 mg/dl and above	High

* Cholesterol levels are measured in milligrams (mg) of cholesterol per deciliter (dl) of blood.

LDL Cholesterol Number	Category
Less than 100 mg/dl	Optimal
100–129 mg/dl	Near optimal/above optimal
130–159 mg/dl	Borderline high
160–189 mg/dl	High
190 mg/dl and above	Very high

HDL Number Affect on Heart Disease Risk

Less than 40 mg/dl	Increases risk
40–59	The higher your HDL, the better
60 mg/dl or higher	Helps lower risk

> **True or false:** Cholesterol supplies you with lots of calories.
> **False.** Cholesterol provides no calories at all. Why? Because you can't break down cholesterol as you do carbohydrates, protein, and fat, so you don't get any energy from it.

The National Cholesterol Education Program Cholesterol Guidelines for Diabetics

	Low	Borderline	High
LDL	less than 100	100–129	130 or higher
HDL	greater than 45	35–45	less than 35
Triglycerides	less than 200	200–399	400 or higher

Heart Disease Risk: Triglycerides

Triglycerides are stored blood fats, and their levels fluctuate throughout the day. High-fat or excessively high-carbohydrate meals, excessive amounts of alcohol, sickness, and stress can all raise triglyceride levels.

If you have elevated triglycerides, you want to pay attention to them because they won't go away by themselves. An excess of these blood fats may be a cause of coronary heart disease. They may also be a consequence of untreated diabetes. What can you do to lower triglycerides in your blood?

▶ Work on your weight if you are overweight or obese
▶ Reduce your intake of saturated fat and cholesterol
▶ Increase your consumption of monounsaturated and polyunsaturated fats
▶ Significantly reduce your alcohol intake

▶ Avoid simple sugars (soda, candy, etc.) and eat moderate portions of all other carbohydrates

▶ Eat more foods containing omega-3 fats

▶ Be physically active 30 minutes or more every day if possible

▶ Control your blood pressure

▶ Avoid smoking

Triglyiceride Number	Category
Less than 150 mg/dl*	Normal
150–199	Borderline high
200–499	High
500 or higher	Very high

* Triglyceride levels are measured in milligrams (mg) of triglycerides per deciliter (dl) of blood.

Nothing you haven't already heard from your doctor, right? That's because all of these suggestions add up to the best type of lifestyle to promote overall health, whether for reducing cardiac or cancer risks, lowering your cholesterol or blood pressure, losing weight or simply improving general well-being!

Heart-Health Strategy #3: Lower High Blood Pressure

Your blood pressure is normal if your numbers are less than 120/80 (or below 130/80 if you have diabetes). To lower your blood pressure, try these techniques:

Achieve and maintain a healthy weight. Overweight people are at greater risk for developing high blood pressure.

Become more physically active. Exercise not only can help you avoid high pressure altogether, it can also help you lower it if you already have the condition. Try to accumulate a minimum of 30 minutes every day if possible. Be sure to check with your doctor first if you haven't exercised for awhile or want to start an exercise program.

Eat a balanced diet loaded with tricklers. Because they are high in nutrients, including fiber, low-GI foods such as fruits, vegetables, and whole grains can help keep your blood pressure in check.

Choose and prepare foods with less salt. If you have high blood pressure or are salt sensitive, you can reduce your risk for heart disease by following the American Heart Association's recommendation to limit your salt intake to no more than $1^{1}/_{4}$ teaspoon or 3 grams of sodium a day. This limit includes the sodium content already *in* the foods.

Drink alcoholic beverages in moderation. Drinking too much alcohol can cause blood pressure levels to rise, whether you actually suffer from high blood pressure or not. So be good to yourself and drink only in moderation.

Heart-Health Strategy #4:
Control Diabetes

Scientists have identified diabetes as an independent risk factor for heart disease; that is, even if you don't have any other risk factors, you're still in danger of developing heart disease simply because you have diabetes. (I explain an associated problem, the Metabolic Syndrome, at length on pages 93–94.) To find out if you have diabetes, and to treat it properly if you do, follow these guidelines:

Get tested. See your doctor, get the prescribed lab work done, and discuss the results with him/her. Diagnostic tests used include:

▶ urine testing for glucose and ketones
▶ blood testing for glucose levels in a fasting state or randomly throughout the day

Prioritize your medical concerns. Are your blood sugars too high? Maybe your LDL cholesterol is off the charts? Are you overweight? Whatever concerns you may have, decide with your doctor which you should tackle first.

Work with your doctor , a certified diabetes educator, and a registered dietitian. These health professionals will help you develop a game plan to address your needs. Chances are, you'll receive a meal plan or new eating strategies that will improve your diet-related risk factors. And guess which type of diet works best? You guessed it: A balanced, high-carb, low-GI diet, with appropriate amounts of heart-healthful proteins and fats. A steady balanced diet of these kinds of healthful foods have been proven to lower cholesterol, lower blood glucose, and promote gradual weight loss, which also improves blood pressure.

Start exercising. There's no need to do anything special; walking is fine. After all, you need no special equipment, and you can do it anytime, anywhere. If you haven't exercised for awhile or want to start an exercise program, always check with your doctor first. That's especially important advice if you have diabetes, because your doctor may have special instructions.

Can You Count to 10,000?

In 2001, U.S. Surgeon General Dr. David Satcher challenged Americans to add on 30 minutes of physical exercise to their normal daily activities. He was echoing the concerns of his predecessor, Dr. C. Everett Koop about the increasing health problems resulting from overweight and obesity. Since then, the Centers for Disease Control and Prevention (CDC) and other health organizations have been encouraging Americans to become more physically active to improve their health.

What does it really take to "become more physically active to improve health?" Really nothing more than a daily walk, which can be as short as going to your colleague's desk instead of sending an e-mail message or as delightful as a trip around the pond after lunch or dinner! If you're an average American, the steps that you automatically take in the course of your day add up to ½ to 1½ miles (900–3,000 steps). Well, if you could consciously add some more steps into your day, **you would become more physically active**. Parking a little further from the door, walking to the post office, walking the kids to the school bus stop, bringing something upstairs when it's in your hand instead of forming a pile for later—these are all painless ways of becoming more physically active.

The goal is to reach 10,000 steps every day. That's five painless miles! You don't need special equipment, or a costly gym membership. You already know how to perform this exercise. And you can do it here and there throughout your day—you don't have to set aside time to exercise, you're already doing it as you go about your day! (Remember Rose in chapter 5?) And you're not starting from zero but from maybe 1,000 or 2,000. And even if you never reach 10,000 steps a day, if your activity increases at all, you're working on improving your health. *Aim for progress, not perfection.*

How do you calculate your steps? The easiest way is to purchase a step-counting pedometer. It is inexpensive and easily found in discount variety or sporting goods stores. Instructions for use are simple. Here are a few suppliers you can check out on the Web:

> www.walk4life.com
> www.new-lifestyles.com
> www.shapeup.org/10000steps.html
> www.thepedometercompany.com/pedometers.html
> www.accusplit.com

There are also Web-based programs you could join. Visit these Web sites for more information:

> www.diabetesincontrol.com/programs/steps/index.shtml
> http://store.diabetes.org

The focus is on improving one's personal best. *Aim for progress, not perfection.* Motivation and commitment can quickly become the driving force behind this chosen lifestyle change. That's exactly what happened recently to one of my patients. Here is his simple story:

How to Aim for Progress not Perfection: Joe's Story

When I first met Joe he was forty-one and newly diagnosed with diabetes. He worked as a civil servant for his local government, as a firefighter for twenty-three years and, more recently, as an administrator, which required less physical activity. He couldn't move around very well since he weighed close to 500 pounds.

Joe's doctor did not think he needed medication for his diabetes; he believed that a change in Joe's eating and exercising habits would probably do the trick.

Upon analysis, Joe's weekday diet consisted of about 2,000 calories. He wasn't a big fruit or vegetable or milk consumer, was prone to eating gusher carbs, and fat contributed close to half of his daily caloric intake. Weekends included eating out, with no self-imposed restrictions on menu choices.

Joe's exercise routine consisted of playing golf a few times a week in the summer. Sometimes he would walk, other times he would use a cart to get from hole to hole.

I agreed with the doctor that diet and exercise could really make a huge difference in Joe's obesity and diabetes. My challenge was to guide him to those changes he felt ready to make and then help him actually make them by providing practical strategies and tips. (This is a wonderful concept we use in diabetes self-management education called the "Patient Empowerment Model.")

I explained about gushers and tricklers and how they affected energy levels and weight. Joe was amazed to learn that he could get off his current glucose roller-coaster ride by constructing meals and snacks that provided adequate energy that the body could sustain over several hours. *I had his attention.* And as he started thinking that finally he might have some real energy, he was looking for a way to make deliberate exercise a part of his new healthy lifestyle.

Joe decided to attack his diet by bringing a baggie of vegetables and two pieces of fruit to work everyday. These foods either accompanied his lunch or he snacked on them throughout the day. He also felt he wanted to give himself more time in the morning to enjoy a calm breakfast, rather than eating and running out the door or eating something in the car. Joe felt these changes were very doable (after all, *he* proposed them) and was eager to begin.

Joe wanted to begin walking more. He thought he'd stay at the municipal building where he worked an extra half hour four times a week and walk on the treadmill that was there. I introduced him to the 10,000-Steps Program. He purchased a pedometer right away and started counting his daily steps.

Are you ready for his results?

Initial pedometer reading: 3,000 steps (1½ miles)

Current pedometer reading: 12,000 steps on a "bad" day (6 miles)

            18,000–20,000 steps 3–4 days/week (9–10 miles)

Initial weight: We're not sure; I could not weigh him on my scale, which weighs up to 450 pounds. From prior weigh-ins, Joe told me he believed he was close to 500 pounds.

Current weight: 420 pounds

Initial mean glucose reading: 159

Current mean glucose reading: 126

All of these changes occurred in just ten months. Joe's doctor continues to see no reason for medication. He just encourages Joe to "keep doing whatever you're doing." If this isn't progress, *what is*?

Do You Have the Metabolic Syndrome?

The Metabolic Syndrome describes a cluster of heart disease risk factors. Experts believe that insulin resistance is at the root of this very serious health concern. Obesity and inactivity promote insulin resistance, a worrisome connection, given our current overfed and underactive American lifestyle. Here is how to tell if you might have the Metabolic Syndrome:

Abdominal Obesity (waist measurement in inches):

Men	greater than 40
Women	greater than 35

Triglycerides	150 mg/dl or higher
HDL Cholesterol	
Men	less than 40 mg/dl
Women	less than 50 mg/dl
Blood Pressure	130/85 mg/Hg or higher
Fasting Glucose	110 mg/dl or higher

For several years, this cluster of risk factors was called Syndrome X because doctors didn't clearly understand what was happening in people with these characteristics. It was a hot topic among endocrinologists, doctors who specialize in metabolic diseases. Current research has shown that Syndrome X is, in fact, a genetic metabolic disorder that puts a person at high risk for coronary heart disease. So now it has become a hot topic for cardiologists too. In fact, medical professionals now carefully monitor a growing number of patients who exhibit this cluster of symptoms: last count: 40 million!

Here's what is going on: If you're insulin resistant, your pancreas secretes enough insulin to meet your body's glucose load, but your cells are uncooperative or resistant to the insulin. So as glucose keeps pouring into your blood from the food that you're digesting, your pancreas just keeps secreting more and more insulin. All this extra insulin manages to keep blood-glucose levels within the normal range, but usually at the high end of normal.

Insulin resistance by itself does not cause diabetes, although some people with diabetes are also insulin resistant (witness Babs in chapter 6). But insulin resistance does lead to chronically high insulin levels. And those high insulin levels lead to high triglycerides, low HDL (good) cholesterol, and high blood pressure—all known risk factors for heart disease.

The good news: Studies have shown that certain types of carbohydrates (yes, the tricklers) increase insulin sensitivity, which decreases insulin resistance.

And This Just In . . .

New research shows that chronic sleep deprivation may contribute to insulin resistance. So how much sleep do you need? More than six and a half hours each night.

Heart-Health Strategy #5: Lose Weight

You already know that diets don't work. Here's a rundown of some of the changes to make to take off that extra weight, reduce your risk of heart disease, and look and feel great at the same time.

Modify your diet. Gradually positive changes will become habits that will last a lifetime. And these habits will be based on improving your health, not losing weight. *Aim for progress, not perfection.* You will see; your extra weight will start to disappear.

Eat three balanced meals a day. Eating three appropriately portioned meals and one to three snacks during the day will keep you from getting too hungry by keeping your blood-glucose levels relatively constant.

Don't drastically cut calories. Most women can lose weight eating 1,400 calories a day; most men, eating 1,700 to 1,800 calories spread throughout the day.

Heart-Health Strategy #6:
Eat More Trickler Carbs as Part of a Balanced Diet

One of the easiest and most heart-healthful lifestyle changes that you can make is to incorporate more slowly digested carbs into your daily diet. This change ties in with the other heart-health strategies too, so you can address several of them at once. Trickler carbs include whole-grain cereals, breads, and crackers, minimally processed flours and other starches, as well as most fruits and vegetables.

The remaining foods that you eat should be lean protein and heart-healthy fats. You can refer back to the Food Guide Pyramid for recommendations by turning to page 6.

In addition, a heart-friendly balanced diet will be low in saturated fat and cholesterol. Limiting these dietary fats will make a huge dent in lowering your LDL cholesterol and help prevent hardening of the arteries from plaque buildup. That means limiting your portions of high-fat foods, including but not limited to, fatty or greasy meats, butter, cream sauces and gravies, bakery products, deep-fried foods, non-fat-reduced cheese, and whole-milk products. Keep in mind that you don't have to stop eating these foods completely—no food is bad—just eat smaller portions, and have them less often.

A heart-healthful balanced diet will also be high in fiber. Fiber in your gut helps to lower LDL cholesterol and triglycerides. Which foods are high in fiber? Carbohydrates such as whole-grain breads and cereals, fruits, and vegetables. There are your tricklers again!

Scientific Proof: Low-GI Carbs Reduce Cardiac Risk Factors

Initial research, dating back as far as 1985, supports the beneficial relationship between low-GI carbs and their ability to lower cholesterol and triglyceride levels in the blood. The astounding results, a drop of 9 to 36 percent, were achieved by replacing about half of the subjects' carbohydrate intake from conventional starches (refined wheat breads, potatoes, highly processed breakfast cereals) to low-GI starches (rye breads, oat bran, bulgur, beans, barley, and spaghetti). The time frame for this study and several others that followed was one month, which means the body is capable of responding this way in a very short period of time. I hope you find this information as motivating as I!

That first study was only the beginning. If you do a Web search on low-glycemic-index research and implications for heart disease you will find 6,390 responses! But let's fast-forward to June 2000. A very large study was undertaken which also confirmed the heart-health benefits of slowly digested tricklers. The results came from the famous Nurses' Health Study, which has been tracking the medical histories and lifestyles of more than 120,000 women since 1976. This particular study looked at how the type of carbohydrates that 75,000 people consumed affected their risk for coronary heart disease. The researchers were comparing high- and low-GI carbs, in other words, gushers and tricklers.

After looking at thousands of food questionnaires, the investigators found that surges of glucose into the blood (from the digestion of refined carbohydrates) increased the risk of coronary heart disease, especially in overweight people.

Even more recently, the *British Journal of Nutrition* published a report in 2003 indicating that a high-glycemic-index diet was one of several factors that is likely to increase post-meal insulin resistance over time. Insulin resistance, we know, is a confirmed risk factor for heart disease, our nation's #1 killer.

These findings have brought into question the soundness of what scientists have been recommending for years: that to reduce heart disease risk, you should eat a low-fat, high-carbohydrate diet. These new findings, along with the knowledge that too much circulating insulin can have a negative impact on heart health, should encourage health authorities to spell out the *type* of carbohydrates we should be eating. Here's what a more precise dietary recommendation for heart health might look like:

"Eat a balanced diet that consists of *high-fiber, slowly digested carbohydrates* with a low to moderate amount of fat, in which saturated fat and cholesterol are minimal and monounsaturated and polyunsaturated fats are eaten in moderation."

Heart-Health Strategy #7: Stop Smoking

Smoking raises your blood pressure and heart rate, lowers levels of good cholesterol, and increases your risk of developing blood clots that can lead to a heart attack. Worse yet, according to the American Heart Association, smoking is the biggest risk factor for sudden cardiac death. To help you kick the habit, try these tips:

Talk to your doctor. From patches to gums to medication, your doctor has lots of options to offer you.

Join a smoking cessation support group. That extra help and support may be just what you need to quit smoking for good.

Don't fear weight gain. Sure, you burn slightly fewer calories at rest once the nicotine leaves your system. But most of the weight comes from what you put in your mouth *in place of* the cigarette—candy, cookies, chocolates, crackers, plain bagels—all gushers, which just make you eat more! So start eating trickler foods *now* to prevent weight gain when you decide to quit smoking.

Shed the Expense

Instead of spending four dollars on cigarettes, why not buy yourself flowers or a half-pound of decaf gourmet coffee?

Heart-Health Strategy #8: Become More Physically Active

As busy as we all are, sometimes it's hard to find enough time to exercise or stay motivated to keep at it. To help you out, here are some exercise tips, many of them from the President's Council on Physical Fitness and Sports:

Check with your doctor first. If you're just starting an exercise program or haven't been active for awhile, get your doctor's okay first to be sure it's safe.

Make exercise a part of your daily routine. Set a regular time to exercise each day and stick to it. If you have workout time written on your calendar, you'll be more likely to keep the "appointment."

Start gradually. Start out slowly—about five to ten minutes at first; then increase your time to thirty to sixty minutes.

Invite a friend to join you. You'll be more likely to exercise regularly if you work out with a friend.

Rest when you need to. You aren't competing with anyone; you're exercising to stay healthy. So take a break when you need it. But if you've been exercising vigorously, don't stop suddenly or you may feel dizzy or faint.

Drink lots of water. Be sure to drink lots of water before, during, and after you exercise. Don't wait until you're thirsty.

Keep a daily written record of your progress. Tracking your progress, whether it's miles walked or time spent lifting weights, can work motivational miracles.

Exercise to your favorite music. Dance around the living room or take a walk with your personal tape player. (Keep the volume low enough, though, that you can hear all the sounds around you.)

Look for distraction. If you really don't like to exercise, ride a stationary bike, walk on a treadmill, or lift weights while watching your favorite TV show or movie. Before you know it, your time will be up! Jack La Lanne has admitted that he has never liked exercise—but he's still doing it at age ninety!

Wear comfy clothing. The more comfortable you are, the more likely you are to enjoy physical activity.

Heart-Health Strategy #9: Manage Stress

Seems like we're rushing around all day, every day—from work meetings to after-work meetings, to kids' soccer practice and music lessons. Leading a stress-free life seems like an impossible dream. Luckily, there are some things you can do to *manage* the stress you have. Here are a few tips:

Accept that stress exists. You may find it comforting to realize that stress is just a part of life and that we're all in the same boat.

Name your stress. Giving your stress a name—whether it's your work schedule, family problems, medical worries, being overweight, or caring for an elderly parent—can help you better identify the problem and find solutions.

Identify your control. Try to determine which stresses you can do something about and look for ways to break down larger problems into several little ones that you can control. Then tackle your concerns one at a time.

Build a support network. You don't have to go it alone. Call on friends and family members to help you through tough times or just to listen. And keep in mind that some stresses may require professional help.

Eat trickler carbs. These slowly digested foods will keep you off the sugar roller-coaster and help you to feel energetic instead of drained. When you feel peppier, you'll also feel more in control and have a better sense of well-being.

Low Saturated Fat
+ Low GI Carbs
Heart Health

Here's the rundown of how to eat for optimum heart health:

▶ Eat a well-balanced diet.
▶ Eat 50 to 60 percent of total daily calories from carbo-hydrate foods.
▶ Make most carbohydrate choices the slowly-digested, low-GI trickler kind.
▶ Limit fat calories to 25 to 35 percent of total calories.
▶ Reduce your daily intake of saturated fat to less than 7 percent of total calories.
▶ Make most of the fats you eat polyunsaturated and monounsaturated.
▶ Consume less than 200 milligrams of cholesterol per 1,000 calories a day.
▶ Gradually increase your fiber intake to 20 to 30 grams a day.

True Stories
from the Healthy Hearts Club

Marty's Story

Marty is a fifty-six-year-old full-time college professor. He is 5'9" and weighs 237 pounds (BMI of 35, or moderately obese). Divorced for the past fifteen years, Marty lives alone and faithfully incorporates a twenty-minute walk into his daily routine; he also tries to play basketball once or twice a week. Marty skips breakfast during the week and picks up lunch between classes. He prepares many of his evening meals at home. When he was forty-three, Marty had a heart attack. Since placing him on cholesterol-lowering medication, his cardiologist has been pleased with the results of Marty's annual blood work. During his last physical, however, Marty's blood pressure was slightly elevated and his fasting blood sugar was above normal.

Marty's Diet: Before Carb Counseling

Breakfast: Four mugs regular black coffee (between 6 and 10 AM)

Lunch: Hamburger, medium fries, diet Coke

Snack: Diet Coke

Dinner: Twelve-oz. steak, half a restaurant portion of fettuccine alfredo, salad, water

Marty's diet made him a second heart attack waiting to happen. He eats too many calories (about 2,600 a day), and his diet is too high in fats and sodium and too low in fiber. Worse yet, Marty typically eats at least half of his calories late in the evening. His unhealthy dietary habits just couldn't be offset by his daily twenty-minute walk and the occasional basketball game. His meals lack the three nutrient heavyweights: fruits, vegetables, and low-fat dairy foods. His elevated blood pressure and moderate obesity are directly affected by the way he eats.

Marty proves that cholesterol-lowering medication isn't the complete remedy for heart health; he needs to make some lifestyle changes too, such as improving his diet, getting more exercise, and managing his stress.

Marty says that he's never hungry, probably because of all the fat he eats—about 1,500 calories worth on an average day. He knows his diet is unhealthful, but he doesn't know how to change it.

How Could Marty Improve His Diet?

To start eating a more healthful and more balanced diet, Marty could eat a breakfast that consists of a low-GI whole-grain bread or cereal, nonfat milk, and fruit. A turkey sandwich on rye with a salad and a piece of fruit would be easy to find in the cafeteria, he admitted. His new rule-of-thumb for dinner, whether at home or eating out, could be to fill half of his plate with vegetables; then his portions of starch and protein, the foods with more calories, would be controlled automatically.

Marty's Diet: After Carb Counseling

Breakfast: Half a pumpernickel bagel with natural, no-salt-added peanut butter and all-fruit jelly, 1 mug of coffee

Snack: A bowl of Special K with a cup skim milk, ¼ cantaloupe

Lunch (brought from home): Reduced-fat cheese and roasted pepper sandwich on rye, pear, water

Snack (two to three times a week): No-sugar-added hot chocolate, 2 oatmeal cookies

Dinner: One cup steamed brown rice, 2 cups steamed vegetables, small grilled chicken breast, water

Snack: Handful of grapes

Seems like a lot of food, doesn't it? Would you believe that Marty's new diet contains about 750 *fewer* calories than before? He also cut his fat intake by 70 percent!

Marty's New Diet Serves Up Success

Marty actually liked eating this new way and found it easy to make the changes. And his results speak for themselves: After six months, he had lost twenty-three pounds! (Ten percent of his body weight—the 10% Solution.) In addition to playing basketball once or twice a week, he started playing golf and softball, and also found time to walk on his treadmill every day. As a result of these changes, his blood pressure is now normal, and his fasting blood-glucose level has dropped 35 percent, putting it back in the normal range.

Will Marty continue to eat heart-healthy meals and exercise? Here's his answer: "Eating low-fat, high-fiber meals isn't hard to do at all. Not only do I feel good, but also my doctor tells me to keep at it, because the changes are working. I can do that!"

Marco's Story

Marco provides another example of how changes can become habits that turn into a healthy lifestyle. Marco, a fifty-six-year-old man of Hispanic descent, works full-time for a news agency. He is 5'9" and weighs 232 pounds (BMI of 34, mildly obese). At fifty-four, he was diagnosed with type 2 diabetes, which he controlled by taking two pills a day. He also has mildly elevated blood pressure, which no medication seemed able to improve. His most recent blood work showed that he has elevated cholesterol. A nonsmoker who occasionally drinks a glass of wine with dinner, Marco tries to walk a mile around his complex three times a week, which takes him twenty minutes. He complains of feeling tired and hungry most days.

Marco's Diet: Before Carb Counseling
Breakfast: Four cups regular coffee with 2% milk, bagel with cream cheese

Lunch: Tuna salad on rye, Manhattan clam chowder, a few saltines, diet Pepsi

Snacks (throughout the day): Chips, cookies, pretzels, diet iced tea

Dinner: Pot roast, pan-fried potatoes, steamed broccoli, escarole sautéed in olive oil, tomato and onion salad, blue cheese dressing, glass of wine

Marco's meals sound fairly typical: They're full of calories and loaded with fat. This high-fat eating style contributed to his mild obesity, and his excess weight negatively affected his diabetes, cholesterol, and blood pressure. And to make matters worse, Marco spent his day on caffeine overload. His twenty-minute walk every other day was a step in the right direction, but only a small one.

How Could Marco Improve His Diet?
A close look at Marco's diet shows that he was eating only about 30 percent of his daily calories from carbohydrates, and the carbs he chose had high-GI values: bagels, saltines, potatoes, pretzels. Along with the steady flow of caffeine (from coffee, diet Pepsi, and diet iced tea), these gusher carbs elevated his blood sugar and stimulated his appetite. If he can start choosing whole-grain breads and crackers and some lower-GI cooked grains such as

pasta or long-grain rice, and if he can reduce his caffeine intake, he'll start feeling more satisfied with fewer calories. Over time his blood sugar, cholesterol, blood pressure, and weight should all go down. He'll also have a lot more energy.

Marco's Diet: After Carb Counseling

Breakfast: Bowl of All-Bran with Extra Fiber, one cup skim milk, a Granny Smith apple, decaf coffee

Lunch: Large garden salad with grilled chicken breast, low-fat balsamic vinaigrette dressing, one pita bread, dish fresh strawberries, sparkling water

Snack: A handful of sourdough pretzel nuggets

Dinner: Two tilapia filets poached in white wine, ear of corn, steamed asparagus, tomato and onion salad with grated cheese, oil, and vinegar, small bunch red grapes, decaf diet soda

Marco's Small Changes Yield Big Results

After just five months of a few diet and exercise changes, Marco lost 25 pounds—enough that his doctor was able to discontinue all his diabetes and blood pressure medications, since his levels had returned to normal. After eighteen months, Marco continued to maintain his new weight of 209 pounds, which is down 23 pounds from his original weight, and slightly more than 10 percent of his total weight. His blood sugar, blood pressure, and cholesterol values stayed normal—all without prescribed medications. Truly, Marco has followed Hippocrates' advice: "Let thy food be thy medicine." This is what he thinks of himself now: "It's unbelievable how good I feel. Not only am I walking every day, but also I jog half the way! I've never had so much stamina!"

THE BOTTOM LINE

➤ Heart disease is the number one killer of American men and women. But if you control your risk factors, it doesn't have to kill you.

➤ You can reduce your risk of heart disease and high blood pressure by eating a balanced diet loaded with trickler carbs, heart-healthful proteins and fats.

➤ To reduce heart attack risk you should also:
  - lower your blood pressure if it's high
  - reduce levels of total and LDL cholesterol
  - increase HDL cholesterol
  - lose weight if you're overweight
  - find out if you have diabetes and control it if you do
  - quit smoking
  - exercise for at least 30 minutes every day
  - manage stress

➤ A healthful diet comes from healthful eating habits. You may still need medication to manage your heart disease risk factors, but why not help yourself by letting food also serve as your medicine?

8

GOOD CARBS FOR KIDS

They may sometimes act older than their years, but when it comes to nutritional requirements, *children are not little adults.* Kids have unique caloric and nutritional needs that change as they grow. They also view food differently than adults do: Whether a food is healthful or not has absolutely no bearing on whether they'll eat it. And kids may ignore hunger pangs if they're having more fun playing with a friend or riding their bikes. But food, especially nutrient-dense food, is essential to kids' health and normal development.

Yet as important as diet is to a child's growth, it seems that many kids are missing out on the healthy diets that their bodies require. Here's the proof:

- Fifteen percent of all U.S. children ages six to nineteen years are overweight.
- In the last 30 years the incidence of overweight children has doubled for ages 6 to 11 and tripled for 12- to 17-year-olds.
- Only 1 percent of school-aged children meet the Food Guide Pyramid serving recommendations for all five major food groups. Sixteen percent of children met none of the recommendations.
- About 10 percent of adolescents aged twelve to nineteen have elevated cholesterol.
- Eight to 45 percent of children and teens with diabetes have type 2; prior to 1999, only 1 to 2 percent had type 2.

These numbers reflect the weight status of *American children.* These statistics scream to parents, doctors, teachers, school boards, and community and government leaders to *do something* to help our kids!

That All-Important First Year

Infants grow faster during their first year of life than at any other time, so their energy requirements are enormous. A healthy baby's birth weight will double in about the first four months of life and triple by the first year. Babies get the energy and nutrients for this fast growth from their food—breast milk or enriched formula and eventually baby food. Because babies are small, they need small quantities of food. But as the data below clearly show, based on their body weight, babies need about triple the calories that a grown man needs! And to promote healthy growth, those calories should be nutrient-packed and balanced.

> **Did You Know . . .** that an adult man weighing 175 pounds can meet his nutritional needs by eating 2,400 calories a day? That breaks down to about 14 calories per pound of body weight. But a four-month-old infant weighing 14 pounds needs about 630 calories a day, or about 45 calories per pound of body weight. (If that 175-pound man ate according to an infant's needs, he'd consume close to 8,000 calories every day!)

Babies Need Fat

> Infants under two years of age need adequate fat in their diets to grow properly—that's why caregivers should feed these babies whole milk, not low-fat or skim.

Growing Bodies Need More Calories

As babies grow into toddlers, small children, and then school-age children, their energy and nutrient needs naturally grow with them. For example, one-year-old children require about 1,000 calories a day, and by age ten, their energy needs jump to 2,000 calories a day. Parents can best meet their children's energy demands by feeding them a daily diet of nutrient-dense, healthful foods—not a steady diet of *calorie-dense* but *nutrient-empty* foods.

Older Kids—and Food

Adolescents are notorious for eating huge amounts of food. Because boys tend to grow faster (once they start) and develop more lean body mass than girls, their energy needs are especially high. Girls usually start to grow earlier than boys and finish their growth spurt sooner, too. The growth spurts of average adolescent girls last about five years (from ages ten to fifteen); the same growth spurt in adolescent boys takes about seven years (from ages twelve to nineteen). So girls' high energy needs peak earlier and decline faster than their male peers.

Teenagers can develop horrible eating habits that may haunt them long into their adult years: They may skip meals or eat large pizzas late at night; they may be able to "get away with" eating lots of junk food, and empty-calorie meals and snacks while their bodies are using up so much energy to grow. But once growth levels off and energy requirements drop, where will all those extra empty-calorie calories go?

The best way for growing teenagers to meet their daily sky-high nutritional needs is by following the 40-Plus well-balanced diet shown on the Food Pyramid. (See page 5.)

THE FOOD PYRAMID FOR CHILDREN

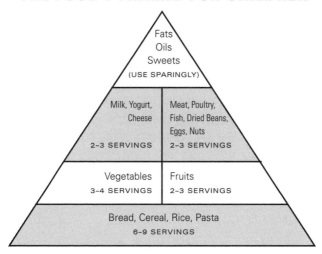

Adapted from *The Glucose Revolution Pocket Guide to Children with Type 1 Diabetes*.
Reprinted courtesy of Marlowe & Company.

Better Nutrition for School Children

The Better Nutrition for School Children Act of 2001, passed by the U.S. Congress, bans the sale or donation to students of soft drinks and other foods of minimal nutritional value, like sugar candies, in schools participating in the National School Lunch Program.

Food: A Kid's Best Friend or Worst Enemy?

Who hasn't seen a young child refuse to eat his peas? Or spinach? Or drink even a small glass of milk? How can a child, you ask yourself, eat macaroni and cheese every single night for dinner and not even consider trying something else? What makes a teenager refuse to bring lunch to school until her best friend starts doing it? There are lots of obstacles that stand in the way of getting good, healthful foods into growing children. Here are a few of them.

Pint-size stomachs. Small children's stomachs fill up fast. So the trick is to get them to eat the most nutritious foods first. That way, they'll get the nutrients they need before getting too full. Little children should be served little portions of a variety of foods; as they grow, food portions should grow along with them.

Picky palates. Children's mouths are very sensitive to temperature, and children also have more taste buds than adults. These differences might explain, then, why children tend to like only a small variety of foods. As they grow, older children usually start liking more diverse flavors, textures, and temperatures. It's a good idea to expose children to a wide variety of foods, though, including vegetables, fruits, and whole-grain breads and cereals; try to make them as interesting, flavorful, and fun to eat as possible, like boat-shaped apple slices or whole-grain peanut-butter and jelly sandwiches cut into cookie shapes. Kids don't care about their health or good nutrition; food has to taste good and be attractive or they won't eat it.

Proof of independence. Children's need to declare their independence can also show up at mealtime. As children mature, these issues begin to fade, especially when parents handle the battles with patience, respect, and understanding.

Peer pressure. All kids want to fit in. And kids will want to eat like their friends and classmates whether in nursery school or college. Unfortunately, the most popular foods are not always the most healthful (in fact, they're almost *never* the most healthful), so this desire to be like everyone else means eating, like everyone else, high-calorie foods with little or no nutritional value. As long as the "junk" foods that children eat at school are offset by healthful meals and snacks at home, there's no real problem. The peer-pressure factor must be given time to run its course.

Now, we can't expect a five-year-old to understand that a daily diet of burgers and fries will potentially, over time, leave plaque deposits on artery walls and possibly lead to a premature heart attack. We know for sure that no teenager looks up the vitamin or mineral content of a food before deciding whether to eat it. But we also know that many young people are teased and suffer real psychological pain because they're overweight. And now more children than ever are being diagnosed with type 2 diabetes—formerly called *adult-onset* diabetes—because of their unhealthful lifestyles. We adults have an obligation to the children in our care to help them foster healthy eating and exercise habits.

The Numbers Tell It All

If you do have a hankering for fast food, it's better to avoid the super-sized meals. (One key to a balanced diet is moderation.) For example, compare these numbers:

Regular (moderate) portions	Super-sized portions
McD burger	Big Xtra! with cheese
Small fries	Super-sized fries
16-oz. Coke	Super-sized Coke
627 calories	**1,805 calories**
19 grams of fat	**84 grams of fat**

Have You Seen *Super Size Me?*

This documentary, released in May 2004 by producer-director-writer-actor Morgan Spurlock, exposes the connection between Americans' entrenched love for fast food and our current woeful health and obesity statistics. Without the approval of his vegan-chef girlfriend and against the consent of his medical advisors, the protagonist films his 30-day exclusive consumption of McDonald's meals, many of which were super-sized servings. As the film concludes, he shares with his viewers the impact his 30-day fast food diet had on his weight, blood pressure, and cholesterol. Can you guess?

Let's Identify the Problems

Kids need to eat a well-balanced diet of adequate, not excessive, calories and be physically active every day. Nothing new, you say. Not exciting, you say. Well, neither is a child who overeats and is inactive and develops type 2 diabetes in middle school. Or kids being unable to play, run, or bike with kindergarten friends because they're obese. Or young people having heart attacks at twenty-one. Unfortunately, these tragic events are happening to more and more children and young adults every day. What's more, experts tell us that this trend shows no signs of reversal.

Do things have to get worse? No. A few dietary and exercise changes can make the difference. After all, our kids have to eat. So why not think of their food as their medicine?

To help zero in on the best ways to improve your child's health, you may ask which is more important, diet (meaning the foods we normally eat) or exercise? If children are tired and overweight, they won't feel very motivated or full of the energy they need to ride a bike or swim. So, in this case, getting the energy from food could make all the difference. And if children sit in front of the TV, eating chips or cookies, as the pounds and problems keep adding up, exercise could really turn things around. So good health includes both *diet and exercise*. Several factors influence children's unhealthy weights: genetics, metabolism, and environment. But, just like adults, kids gain weight when they eat more calories than they burn. So let's take a look at the two major causes of young people's expanding waistlines.

Cause #1: Our children overeat. Why? Because in this country, you can get food everywhere, at any hour of any day. And that food is often cheap and high in fats, sodium, and calories. For example: You pay $4.99 for an Italian hero at a 24-hour convenience store. That one item contains 800 calories and 32 grams of fat!

We live in a culture of portion distortion. If you compare recommendations from the Food Guide Pyramid for daily portions and super-sized meals and snacks, you'll be shocked at the differences. For example, one McDonald's quarter-pounder with cheese, medium fries, and a Coke contains 980 calories, 46 grams fat, 10 teaspoons sugar, and 1,300 mg sodium. That's about 50 percent of the calories, 69 percent of the fat, 80 percent of the sugar, and 57 percent of the sodium that a ten- or twelve-year-old needs *for the whole day*! (And these numbers don't represent super-sized portions.) Try these tips to help your child eat a more balanced diet:

Set a good example. If you want your child to eat a more healthful diet and get more exercise, why not show the way? Prepare meals that are healthful for the whole family and eat them yourself. Keep fruits, vegetables. dry-roasted nuts, and low-fat milk products visible for quick-grab snacks.

Ask your child to help. If you ask them, your kids will probably be thrilled to help you shop and prepare healthful foods and meals. Have them pick out the apples at the supermarket or prepare the salad for dinner. They're more likely to take pride in (and *eat*) a meal in which they've been involved.

Cut fruits and vegetables into finger-food sizes. Presenting healthful foods in an interesting way can make them more fun for small children to eat.

Ask your child to help plan the menu. If your child helps you plan menus, he'll pick foods he enjoys (and you can help guide him toward appropriate choices).

Cause #2: Our kids are inactive. Why? Because carpools take our children to and from school and after-school activities, and parents' and kids' tight schedules don't allow a lot of time for exercise. What's more, kids spend a lot of time watching TV or sitting at the computer (some experts estimate 26 hours or more every week) instead of playing outside. And kids' poor diets and lack of energy make them too tired, too overweight, or too sick-feeling to run and play. Here are some ways to get your child to become more physically active:

Do things as a family. Why not start some new traditions and go for walks or bike rides as a family? Like to do yard work? Make it a game and ask the kids to help. Not only will you all be getting great exercise, you'll be spending time together, too.

Be a role model. If your kids see you gardening, washing the car, raking leaves, and taking evening walks, they'll recognize your good example and be more likely to follow your lead.

Work exercise into every day. Our bodies were built to move, so why not get your child to include more *move*ment throughout the day? After all, walking and climbing stairs don't require special equipment, club memberships, or skills. If you can help make exercise part of your kid's ordinary day, then there's no need to make time for exercise, it's already there!

But if you are looking for some help, here are some TV and video options to choose from:

- Cable television network Nickelodeon's *LazyTown* program
- PBS' *Boohbah* show and related toys
- PlayStation2 EyeToy video game series
- Spider-Man 2 Web Action Gaming System
- DanceDance Revolution video game
- PlayTV wireless video game series
- Several children's exercise videos can be found at www.collagevideo.com

Did You Know . . .

- ➤ that 91 percent of food commercials shown during children's programming advertise foods that are either high-fat, high-sugar, or high-salt?
- ➤ that the American Academy of Pediatrics recommends limiting TV time to a maximum of two hours a day? Research shows that the more a child watches TV, the greater the risk for higher cholesterol levels.

High-Fructose Corn Syrup: A Not-So-Sweet Story

We've all heard about this ingredient or seen it listed on food labels. There is not likely one American citizen of walking age who hasn't tasted this ingredient. Do we know what it is? Where it comes from? How much we actually consume of it? Or what it does inside our bodies?

High-fructose corn syrup (HFCS) is a food additive used to sweeten such foods as soda and soft drinks, candies, cookies, ice cream and many, many other foods, including baby foods. And its presence isn't limited to just sweet-tasting foods: HFCS can also be found in ketchup, hot dog buns, and some varieties of salad dressings, just to name a few others.

HFCS results from the chemical combination of fructose and dextrose (a form of glucose that comes from cornstarch) in almost equal parts. Just like table sugar (which also contains fructose and glucose in equal parts), HFCS, a refined carbo-hydrate (aka gusher carbohydrate in this book—and in your body!) contains four calories per gram (4 grams make up a tea-spoon; therefore, there are 16 calories per teaspoon of HFCS, the same caloric content of sugar). It is the most consumed sweetener in the United States. And since it is 1.5 times sweeter than sugar, a slightly smaller quantity will produce the same degree of sweetness. Why is HFCS used so profusely in the food industry? It's sweeter and less expensive than sugar and has good shelf stability.

Recent research attests to how serious a problem HFCS con-sumption is in this country. Today, it is believed that *20 percent* of our carbs and a full *10 percent* of our total daily calories come from HFCS *alone!* While prior to 1966, the average American had *never consumed* any HFCS, but by 2001 that intake soared to 62.6 pounds! The Sugar Association estimates average sugar con-sumption to be approximately 40 pounds per person per year. This is why the USDA continues to adamantly stress our need to reduce *all added sugar* consumption from our daily average of 31 teaspoons to no more than 10 to 12 teaspoons.

Why such a fuss? There is growing concern that fructose may act more like a fat than a sugar in the body. It may encourage insulin resistance and elevated triglycerides. And there is strong research support for a clear parallel between increases in total and refined carbohydrate calories, like table sugar and especially HFCS, and the current staggering rise in obesity and type 2 diabetes. To cite one example, the prestigious Nurses' Health Study, which has been tracking 122,000 individuals since 1976, has singled out regular soda as a contributor to these two health concerns. We could make a serious dent in our sugar intake by limiting—eliminating would be even better—those foods that we consume with HFCS.

Maybe a good way to start would be to cut in half sweetened beverages, or choose a light or plain yogurt instead of the regular kind. You don't have to turn your eating habits upside-down; just take small but consistent steps towards a new behavioral pattern. *Aim for progress, not perfection.* Here are some other ideas to reduce your sugar intake:

- Recognize "sugar" by all of its names: sucrose, high-fructose corn syrup, corn syrup, dextrose, glucose, fructose, maltose, honey, and molasses.
- Consume less "liquid candy," which is all that regular soft drinks are. Dilute them with seltzer or water or replace them with a quick homemade smoothie (fruit + low-fat milk/yogurt).
- Consider fruit "drinks," "beverages," "ades," or "cocktails" the same as soda without the fizz. Drink water or eat a piece of fruit instead.
- Limit the size and frequency of candy and sweet baked goods like cookies, cakes, pies, doughnuts, and pastries.
- Be cautious of your fat-free snacks. They may contain a lot of added sugar and a lot of calories.
- Choose breakfast cereals that are whole grain (they will have 4 or more grams of fiber per serving) and that have no more than 8 grams of added sugar per serving.

Soda Facts: Tried and True
- A 12-ounce can of regular soda contains approximately 12 teaspoons of added sugar.
- Fifteen billion gallons of soda were sold in the U.S. in 2000. This means every man, woman and child averaged one can every day for the entire year!

➤ Two-year-olds get more sugar from soda than they do from cookies, candy, and ice cream *combined.*

➤ The majority (56 percent) of eight-year-olds drink soft drinks every day.

➤ One out of three teenage boys drinks at least three cans of soda per day.

➤ Kids who drink soft drinks consume about 200 more calories/day than those who don't.

The Rest of the Sugar Story

In chapter 2, I explained about single sugars and double sugars, where they are found in our foods and what the body does with them. Now I've just described what high-fructose corn syrup is, where and why it's found in so many commonly eaten foods, and how it may be affecting your health.

To be thorough, I would like to conclude my sugar story with a mention of the sugar replacers (also called polyols or sugar alcohols) and artificial sweeteners that your gut is likely to encounter on a regular, if not daily, basis.

You've seen ingredients such as sorbitol, xylitol, mannitol, maltitol, lactitol, isomalt and hydrogenated starch hydrolysates in food products like sugarless gum, no-sugar-added frozen desserts, candies, and jams. Or maybe you just skip over them when you're reading the food label because they have weird-sounding names and you don't know what they are anyway. Well, I can't do much about their names but I can tell you that these are all nutritive sweetening agents that the body breaks down differently than sugar. They are absorbed more slowly into the bloodstream from the intestines and they provide just 2 to 3 calories/gram. These characteristics make them all good sweet-food choices when trying to curb caloric intake or regulate blood-glucose levels. They also have a built-in benefit: their potential laxative effect, if over consumed, makes them self-limiting. These sugar replacers, once called sugar alcohols, contain no alcohol at all. The "alcohol" refers to the chemical structure of their molecules.

There are also non-nutritive sugar substitutes: Sweet'n Low (saccharin) comes in the pink packet; Equal (aspartame) comes in the blue packet; Splenda (sucralose) comes in the yellow packet. Choice is based on palate preference. They are calorie-free and do not affect glucose levels in the blood. Stevia, a naturally-occurring plant sweetener, is not found in foods but can be purchased in packets like the other sweeteners. The body recognizes it sweetness but cannot break it down, so there are no calories or glucose elevations attached to the ingestion of stevia. And to complete the list, there are two new artificial sweeteners that will soon enter the market. If you come across "neotame" or "tagatose," that's them!

Spoonfuls of Sugar

1 teaspoon table sugar (sucrose)	15 calories
1 teaspoon brown sugar	16 calories
1 teaspoon fructose	12 calories
1 teaspoon honey	21 calories
1 teaspoon jelly	16 calories
1 packet Sweet'n Low	0 calories
1 packet Equal	0 calories
1 packet Splenda	0 calories

Trickler Carbs to the Rescue

Energy comes from the food we eat. When adults eat a balanced diet that provides consistent amounts of energy throughout the day, they don't feel draggy. In fact, there always seems to be enough energy to keep going. Food works the same way in young bodies. So an energetic child will go to school, participate in some exercise after school (soccer, ballet, swimming), do homework, take part in family chores, and then go to bed—all on the energy that came from that day's breakfast, lunch, dinner, and snacks.

But what *kind* of breakfast, lunch, dinner, and snacks? Nutrient-dense, well-balanced meals and snacks provide the right amount of calories, vitamins, protein, and minerals that growing bodies need to keep going all day long. And low-GI carbs included in these meals and snacks assure that steady supply of energy to enjoy a physically active day.

Trickler carbs work the same in young bodies as they do in older ones. These carbs provide:

▶ Energy that kids need throughout the school day to grow and to concentrate and stay mentally alert. A drifting mind sometimes means a hungry body.

▶ A steady supply of energy that carries over to after-school activities. Sometimes, kids show little interest in extracurricular activities because their blood-glucose levels are low.

▶ A feeling of satisfaction or fullness, preventing kids from eating unnecessary calories. Let's face it: Sometimes kids eat because low blood-glucose levels make them *feel* hungry, not because they've actually run out of food calories to burn for energy.

So, to repeat the most healthful diet prescription for a young, growing body:

Eat a well-balanced diet of adequate, not excessive, calories, *including slowly digested carbohydrates* and be physically active every day.

The Ideal Fiber Formula for Kids: An Easy Numbers Game

Can't figure out how much fiber your child should be eating? Try this:

Take your child's age and add five. That gives you the right daily amount of fiber (in grams) the child should be getting. Secret: As children grow, so should their fiber intake.

Example: Five-year-old's fiber needs: 5 + 5 = 10 grams
Six-year-old's fiber needs: 6 + 5 = 11 grams

Before you know it, your child has developed a healthful habit.

Where Do I Find Fiber?

Looking for good fiber sources for your kids? Here are a few:

Chocolate Applesauce Cupcake (see page 199) = 4 grams

Fiber-High Bran Muffin (see page 153) = 4 grams

Half-cup High-Test Granola (see page 152) = 5 grams

Half-cup Simply Delicious Applesauce (see page 202) = 3 grams)

Pizzetta (see page 196) = 3 grams

2 Cherry-Oat Crunchies (see page 197) = 2 grams

12 oz. Chocolate-Pear Smoothie (see page 201) = 3 grams

A slice of whole-grain bread = 2 or more grams

Medium-sized piece of fruit = 2–4 grams

Small handful peanuts = 2 grams

2 tablespoons peanut butter = 2 grams

Trickler Carbs and Kids

Question: Why do young people have high nutritional needs?

Answer: Because they're growing.

Question: How can caregivers best meet these high nutritional needs?

Answer: By encouraging kids to eat a well-balanced diet that contains a variety of nutrient-dense foods.

Question: What foods are nutrient-dense but not excessively high in calories, yet provide a steady source of energy to help prevent hunger?

Answer: Low-GI carbs.

Is Your Child Overweight?

Wondering whether your child is overweight? Here's how to find out: The next time you visit your pediatrician, ask him/her to plot your child's height and weight on a chart. If your child's percentile for weight is much greater than his percentile for height, that's a warning sign. (That may not hold true, though, for boys in early adolescence, who are about to go through their growth spurts. That's when boys build heavy muscles, which can skew the charts.) Also, any child with a BMI greater than the 95th percentile for age and sex is considered overweight.

Bye-Bye, Baby Fat

The old-fashioned view that baby fat melts off by adolescence just doesn't hold true anymore, because today's kids have developed poor eating and lifestyle habits that prevent baby fat from ever melting! And the statistics prove it. Years ago, when baby fat was reserved just for babies, there was no fast food, no eating out, no computers, and no sitting in front of the TV for hours on end. Now these lifestyle habits continue from childhood into adolescence and beyond, so *baby* fat turns into *adult* fat.

Betsy's Story

Betsy, a second-grader, lives with her parents and younger sibling. Betsy is the only person in her family with a weight problem; she weighs 80 pounds and stands just 3'8"; her weight is off the growth chart. For her height, Betsy is considered severely obese. The pediatrician advised Betsy's mother to talk to a registered dietitian for advice; the goal was for Betsy to lose about eight pounds over the next twelve months (the 10% Solution). Betsy's mom thought this was a great idea: She would learn more about healthy eating for her daughter and the entire family. And so she came to my office.

Betsy's Diet: Before Carb Counseling

Breakfast: Three-quarter cup Rice Chex, 4 oz. 1% milk
Snack: Eight oz. 1% milk, breakfast bar
Lunch: Two ounces turkey breast on small roll, $\frac{1}{2}$ cup instant mashed potatoes with gravy, 8 oz. 1% milk
Snack: Two Oreo cookies, ice cream sandwich
Dinner: A small bowl commercial chicken noodle soup, 5 saltines, cup of orange soda
Snack: Half an orange

Betsy's diet needed lots of changes. For starters, she was eating about 1,700 calories, about 300 more than she needed in a day. And though she drank enough milk to meet the minimal calcium needs of a seven-year-old, on some days she wasn't getting enough high-quality protein foods (from foods such as meat, fish, and eggs). Her fiber intake was low because she ate few fruits, vegetables, and whole grains. Her limited food choices meant that she might not be getting enough vitamins and minerals from her diet. She complained of being too tired to play after school and said she was hungry all the time. Because she was obese at such a young age, Betsy could face weight-related health problems later in life if she doesn't make some changes now.

How Could Betsy Improve Her Diet?

Betsy could start eating better meals by decreasing her starch intake; most of the starches in her diet come from gushers—Rice Chex, instant mashed potatoes, white-flour rolls, cookies, saltines, and soda. For these starches, she could substitute tricklers such as whole-grain cereals, breads, and crackers, and some slowly digested fruits and vegetables. These changes will allow Betsy to eat fewer—yet still enough—calories. What's more, she'll have more energy and feel fuller longer. In the process, she'll be eating balanced meals that meet the demanding nutrient needs of a growing seven-year-old. With her newfound energy, Betsy could look forward to active play time every day after school.

Betsy's Diet: After Carb Counseling

Breakfast: Three-quarter cup Life cereal, 4 oz. 1% milk, $\frac{1}{2}$ cup of strawberries

Snack: Half a sandwich-size bag of green grapes (about 17), 4 oz. 1% milk

Lunch: Ham and reduced-fat-Swiss sandwich, 2 slices rye bread (crusts removed), 6 baby carrots, 4 oz. 1% milk

Snack: A handful of Teddy Grahams, 4 oz. 1% milk

Dinner: Baked chicken drumstick, breaded, without skin, 1/3 cup mashed sweet potato, 1/2 cup steamed green beans with vinaigrette, 1/2 cup of natural applesauce, 4 oz. 1% milk
Snack: Half cup low-fat cooked pudding

Betsy's Back on the Growth Charts

By making small but consistent changes to her diet, Betsy lost seven pounds in eight months. During the end-of-the-year holiday season, her mom thought it would be best to help her maintain that loss, and once the normal school routine started again, they would work at losing that final pound so that she would reach her goal weight. This is exactly what happened. When Betsy returned to her doctor for her annual physical exam, he was pleased with how well he found her; with her eight-pound loss from the prior year, her weight was back on the growth chart again. The doctor encouraged Betsy and her mom to continue with their current dietary program and check back in six months.

Betsy's mom, thrilled that her little girl has more energy and is less moody, is especially pleased that meal and snack times no longer involve mother-daughter battles.

The Perfect School Lunch

We know that there is no one nutritionally complete food. That's why we try to encourage our children to eat a variety of foods from several of the six food groups at each meal. Macaroni and cheese is not a nutritionally complete meal by itself. Neither is a bowl of mashed potatoes, or two pieces of string cheese, or just a yogurt or an apple.

Here is what all young children in school need in their lunchboxes every day:

2 grain servings	=	2 slices whole-grain bread or 1 cup macaroni
2 ounces protein	=	2 oz. chicken or 2 tablespoons peanut butter

1 vegetable serving	=	8 carrot sticks or 1 cup salad
1 fruit serving	=	7 large strawberries, small apple, or 12 large grapes
1 dairy serving	=	8 oz. skim/low fat milk or yogurt
small amount fat	=	small handful nuts, margarine, butter, or mayonnaise

These are not exact portions. Smaller, younger children will need smaller portions, while the calories should increase significantly as children approach pre-adolescence and adolescence. But I want to show you the *composition* of a healthy balanced school lunch. You can adjust the portions as needed. In fact, why not try it tomorrow?

Tom's Story

Tom discovered that he had elevated blood fats when he was a sophomore in high school and just fifteen and a half years old. He carried 143 pounds on a 5'4" body frame, making him overweight. His doctor was concerned about Tom's frightening cholesterol profile: His bad cholesterol was very high, his good cholesterol was low, and his fasting triglyceride levels were also very high. Because there's a strong history of heart disease and diabetes on both sides of Tom's family, and because adolescents aren't usually treated for high cholesterol with medication, Tom's mom hoped that a better diet would be her son's "pill." Tom didn't smoke or drink alcohol; he played tennis once or twice a week and forced himself to walk two miles every day since his most recent doctor's visit. He admitted that he was a fussy eater, willing to eat a very limited variety of acceptable foods, which included two or three types of fruits and vegetables, no ham, no fish, and no cheese, except on pizza.

Tom's diet (summer schedule): Before Carb Counseling

Breakfast (10:30 AM): Three cups Froot Loops, 8 oz. 1% milk

Snack: Eight oz. ginger ale
Lunch: One slice cheese pizza, can Coke
Snack: Eight oz. ginger ale
Dinner: Fried chicken breast (with skin), cucumber and carrot sticks, pickle, 8 oz. ginger ale
Snack: Two or three scoops of sherbet
Snack: An apple, 8 oz. orange juice, 12 oz. 1% chocolate milk

On this kind of a day (and there was little variation in his choices from day to day), Tom consumed about 2,100 calories, which is at the low end of the appropriate range for his daily energy needs. His fat intake (approximately 50 grams) was only about 21 percent of his total calories. But about 40 percent of his total caloric intake came from nutritional "lightweights," such as Froot Loops, soda, and sherbet. These foods gave his body empty calories; that is, his body did all the work of breaking them down into glucose but that's all he got—just glucose, not very many of the 40-Plus nutrients he also needed. His diet lacked fiber and heart-healthy fats and contained a lot of hidden sugar (probably between forty-five and fifty teaspoons!). No wonder he complained of being tired and hungry all the time, didn't feel like playing sports or being physically active during his summer vacation. Tom was on a daily roller-coaster ride of blood-glucose highs and lows.

How Could Tom Improve His Diet?

Wow! Forty-five to fifty teaspoons of sugar in a day gave Tom a *long* roller-coaster ride. His weight gain and high triglyceride levels were no surprise, given the way he was eating and his family's medical history. By agreeing to eat whole-grain cereals and breads, and including more fruits and vegetables throughout the day, Tom would quickly feel more energetic all day long. He would also lose weight gradually, because low-GI foods help you burn fat more readily rather than store it. (See chapter 4 for a detailed explanation). Perhaps most important of all, a low-GI diet would help Tom attack his elevated cholesterol and triglycerides.

Tom's Diet: After Carb Counseling

Breakfast: One and a half cups 100% Bran Flakes, 8 oz. skim Plus milk, water with a multivitamin pill

Lunch: Sandwich (turkey or chicken breast, or fat-free bologna), 2 slices rye bread, cucumber spears, apple, water *or* (on days when he worked at the pizza shop) slice cheese pizza, apple, diet Coke

Dinner: One or two ears corn, grilled chicken breast (no skin), broccoli with olive oil (he loves the way his mom makes this and eats 2 cups), 2 handfuls grapes, water

Snack: Twelve oz. 1% chocolate milk, 2 to 3 fat-free oatmeal cookies

Tom's Energy Surge

Although his new diet plan wasn't ideal, it was a huge improvement. Most important, Tom agreed that he could live with it. After six months of his new lifestyle, Tom's cholesterol dropped 136 points, putting him well within the normal range. The same was true for his LDL (bad) cholesterol, which dropped 98 points; his fasting triglycerides also fell 184 points. In other words, all of his blood values that used to be out of the normal range were now back to normal. Tom lost 19 pounds; he ate fewer *empty* calories, although he was still eating about the same *number* of calories. He also got more exercise (he swam and went bike riding most days). And because he had more energy, he didn't have to force himself into activity. His doctor was amazed at Tom's new blood levels and his mother was relieved that she now had a plan to help her son eat better and improve his health. And Tom was happy that everyone was off his case. He says: "I know I'm still a picky eater, but I think I've done great, and even better, so does my mother!"

THE BOTTOM LINE

➤ Children's nutritional needs are not the same as those of adults.

➤ Kids have unique caloric and nutrient needs that change as they grow.

➤ Infants grow faster during their first year of life than at any other time.

➤ Babies under two years of age need adequate fat in their diet to grow properly.

➤ Like adults, children and young people should eat a well-balanced diet of adequate—not excessive—calories, *including slowly digested carbohydrates* and be physically active every day.

9

GOOD CARBS
FOR PEAK PERFORMANCE

Whether you're sleeping, thinking, eating, singing, or running a marathon, glucose makes you move. And there's a specific relationship between your movements and the source of the energy (carbs) that fuels those movements.

If you look at the parking lot outside an office building or shopping mall, you'll see lots of cars of all different sizes and shapes, makes and colors, capabilities and prices. But they all share one thing in common: they all need fuel to move. And not just any fuel will work in these vehicles. Cars need the fuel they were built to run on—gasoline.

Your body, just like a car, runs on its own preferred fuel—glucose. And the best "pump" from which to get this fuel is dietary carbs. Your body has an easier time extracting energy from carbs than it does from fats or proteins, and so it prefers them.

So when you're thinking about different energy sources for exercise, it's important to know that your body prefers carbs. Because carbohydrates are your body's fuel of choice, it doesn't have to work very hard to get energy from them. And if your body uses a minimal number of calories to break down its energy source (through carb digestion), there will be more calories left to burn during exercise. That extra energy could mean the difference between *finishing* the race and *winning* the race!

From the "Sad but True" File

➤ About 60 percent of American adults are not regularly active, and about 25 percent are not active at all.
➤ Nearly 50 percent of young Americans between the ages of twelve and twenty-one are not regularly active.

> ➤ Less than 50 percent of American students currently partic-
> ipate in physical education classes.
> ➤ Only about 20 percent of American children and adults exer-
> cise regularly.
> ➤ Children of active parents are six times more likely to be
> physically active themselves than children of inactive
> parents.

High Test, High Payback

It may be more costly in the short term, but putting high-test
gasoline in your car has definite advantages. When you give your
car top-notch fuel, it responds with top-notch performance: no
knocks or pings, just a dependable, smooth ride every time. Your
car will likely spend less time in the repair shop too. Over the
years, your car will continue to perform reliably and give you few
headaches. *But to perform its best, you need to give it the right kind
of fuel.*

Likewise, if you give your body the best fuel possible, it, too, will
respond with high performance; it may be high performance in
school, at work, or at home; it may be high performance during a
basketball game, a race, or an intense workout at the gym. It
should come as no surprise to you that the best sources for your
glucose fuel are the carbohydrate foods you eat. Let's review why:

▶ Your body digests the food you eat to get the energy contained in those foods. That energy enables you to do
absolutely everything—from breathing to recovering
from a cold to whistling to white-water rafting.

▶ Just as gasoline makes cars run, glucose makes your
body run.

▶ Your body can extract glucose from other foods, but
carbs are the easiest for it to use.

▶ How do carbs benefit you during exercise? By leaving
you lots of leftover energy after digestion, you have more
energy to use for exercise.

Your body is a machine—just like your car.

Don't Forget Your Water!

You need four to eight ounces of water every fifteen to twenty minutes while you exercise—whether you're thirsty or not. This amount is in addition to the eight to twelve cups of water you should already be drinking every day. But no need to worry: All of the beverages you drink contain water, as do most foods you eat, even foods such as bread, nuts, meat, and cheese; the only foods that don't contain water are vegetable oils. By the way, alcohol and caffeinated beverages aren't good fluid sources; they can lead to dehydration.

Trickler Carbs, Your High-Test Fuel

If you can shift your body into "cruise control," you'll find that your energy will last longer, with plenty of time before the "empty" light starts to flash. Quickly digested carbs rapidly release just-digested energy into your bloodstream, where insulin quickly responds and hurries it to the cells, leaving you with an exhausted energy supply. So if you're starting to exercise, where will your energy come from if your tank is empty before you even start your trip? In contrast, slowly digested tricklers help you go the distance simply because they drip (or trickle) energy into your blood over a long period of time.

Gushers Aren't All Bad

There are certain circumstances when you need gushers; for example: during prolonged exercise, when you don't want your blood-glucose levels to drop too low, and after intense exercise, when you want to speed up glycogen storage, since you used some glycogen during exercise. (Glycogen, you may remember, is your body's quickly available form of stored energy.)

Tony's Story

Tony was a bachelor in his mid-twenties, working as a full-time firefighter, and taking college courses a few nights a week when

I met him. At 5'9" and 189 pounds (BMI of 28), Tony was overweight. (His goal weight would be 170 pounds—the 10% Solution.) Tony has been a serious athlete ever since high school and competes in bi- and triathlons several times a season.

Tony noticed that his performance level had been slipping over the past few competitions and thought that his steady weight gain since high school was part of the problem. He wasn't quite sure how to fix things: He was committed to an intense workout most days, so he knew he was burning a lot of calories; and he was also intensely hungry *all* the time—whether he worked out or not. Could he be overeating, with all the regular exercise he was getting?

Tony's family has a strong history of diabetes, heart disease, and obesity, but Tony thought he was insuring himself against these possible health concerns by getting lots of exercise.

Tony's Workout Schedule

Tony kept to a pretty rigorous training program: Not only did he run four to six times a week, he also bikes three times a week for 90 minutes and weight-trained five to seven times a week for 30 minutes.

Tony's Diet: Before Carb Counseling

> **Breakfast:** Two or 3 cups Rice Chex, 16 oz. 2% milk
> **Snack:** Banana, pear, 2 carrots
> **Lunch:** Two slices white sandwich bread, 3 oz. roast beef, 2 handfuls pretzels, 1 cup strawberries, 32 oz. Gatorade
> **Dinner:** One lb. steak, 1½ cups green beans with approx. 2 tbs. butter, 2 cups linguine, 1 cup cream sauce, 32 oz. Gatorade
> **Late-night snack:** One sleeve saltines, 32 oz. Gatorade

Even though Tony was committed to an intense workout schedule, he was eating way too many calories. On an average day, such as the one above, Tony's food intake could add up to about 5,500 calories and over 200 grams of fat! Even for an athlete, this diet resulted in weight gain—as body fat. And given his family's medical history, Tony's diet was placing him in danger of heart disease and possibly diabetes. Reducing his caloric intake by 50 percent would still meet his daily metabolic requirements and give him the energy he needed for his workouts.

How Could Tony Improve His Diet?

Tony would feel fuller longer if he ate a low-GI cereal in the morning such as Bran Buds or old-fashioned oatmeal instead of Rice Chex. He could also replace his gusher white bread with a whole wheat pita or whole-grain pumpernickel bread. Then he could reduce his food portions at other meals throughout the day. His snacks could consist of light yogurt or low-fat milk, oatmeal, or Social Tea biscuits or some ice cream, fruit, or chips and salsa. And the only time he should have drunk 32 ounces of Gatorade, a quickly digested sugar drink, is on those three days a week when he went on a ninety-minute bike ride. For that long bike ride, Tony might need a handy energy source to replenish his body's emptied glucose and glycogen stores.

Tony's Diet: After Carb Counseling

Breakfast: Two cups oat bran cereal, 12 oz. 1% milk, large apple, water

Snack: One to 2 handfuls of grapes

Lunch: Two slices whole-grain pumpernickel, 3 oz. lean roast beef, 1 tbs. mayonnaise, sandwich-sized bag of raw vegetables (baby carrots, celery, pepper strips), large pear, 2 oatmeal cookies, water

Snack: Low-fat granola bar, 8 oz. 1% milk

Dinner: One and a half cups long-grain rice pilaf, 6 oz. rosemary chicken breast, 2 cups steamed broccoli florets with 2 pats butter and 2 tbs. slivered almonds, water

Snack: Small apple cinnamon muffin (from mix), 8 oz. 1% milk

As you can see, fewer calories don't leave Tony with an empty plate! Yet his new meal plan adds up to 50 percent fewer calories and 70 percent less fat than his old diet. And his meals aren't low-calorie or low-fat; they're just not the excessive quantities that as they once were.

Tony's New Competitive Edge

In the first five weeks of his new way of eating, Tony dropped seven and a half pounds. Then, after ten weeks, he reached his goal of 170 pounds. In his first competition at his new weight, a biathlon, he finished 66th out of 200-plus competitors, his personal best. Tony told me, "I never dreamed I could run so fast or bike so long on half the calories I was used to eating!"

Eight years have passed since Tony first began incorporating low-GI carbs into his meal and snack planning. He has long since completed his college courses but is still a full-time firefighter, still an elite-level athlete, and alas! still an unattached bachelor. To date he has competed in four Iron Man Competitions, placing in the *top 2 percent* in his age category for men in America! He is currently taking a year off from racing but that doesn't mean Tony has stopped exercising. In addition to running six miles four times a week (average running time: 42 minutes), he has undertaken a serious resistance training regimen. As a result of this new focus, Tony has added on about ten pounds of muscle. He is still wearing the same pants size, but when his suit jackets kept ripping at the seams, he realized his upper body had expanded two sizes! At his last physical at the firehouse, his body fat was measured at an all-time low of 11.5 percent. And all of the medical visits and blood work results to date continue to show no signs of any looming health problems—the best part of this success story.

His "rest year" nearly complete, Tony is starting to gear up for his intense triathlon training schedule again. "Your counseling changed my life. I believe 50 to 70 percent of my athletic success is due to my low-GI way of eating."

What is the Iron Man?

An Iron Man competition consists of: 2.4-mile swim, immediately followed by 112-mile bike ride, immediately followed by a marathon run (26.2 miles). Contestants are given 17 hours to complete all three sections of the race. **Tony has never needed more than 11.5 hours.**

Here are some Web sites for more information:

www.usatriatholon.org

www.triathelete.com

Reaching the Finish Line

Low-GI carbohydrates provide you with a slow, steady flow of energy that lasts for a prolonged period of time. What's more, these foods don't cause blood glucose highs and lows; tricklers offer no roller-coaster rides—just smooth, consistent rides in cruise control.

Whether it's for peak performance or just to improve a workout or physical skill (such as playing tennis or skiing), training is an essential part of exercise: Practice makes perfect. But efficient fueling is just as crucial. In fact, for some people it may just provide that elusive competitive edge.

THE BOTTOM LINE

➤ Your body, just like a car, "runs" on its own preferred fuel—glucose. The best fuels are dietary carbs that your body digests slowly.

➤ Your body has an easier time extracting energy from carbs than it does from fats or proteins. That leaves you with more leftover energy for exercise.

➤ Gusher foods come in handy when you don't want your blood-glucose levels to drop too low and when you want to speed up glycogen storage.

➤ Low-GI carbohydrates provide you with a slow, steady flow of energy for a prolonged period of time.

➤ Make sure you drink enough fluids throughout the day.

10

CHOOSE THE RIGHT CARBS
FOR YOU

If there's a message to take home from this book, it's that you should eat a balanced diet that consists of a variety of high-fiber, slowly digested carbohydrates, and heart-healthful proteins and fats. How do you transfer this information from your head onto your plate or into a brown bag? And how can you recognize the best choices on a menu or supermarket shelf?

Maybe the following lists will help: I've provided three breakfast, lunch, and dinner examples, along with a wide variety of snacks. The average nutrient breakdown for these meals (excluding snacks) is 54 percent carbohydrate, 22 percent protein, and 24 percent fat.

Please keep this in mind: The portions of some foods (such as sandwich fillings, pasta, and chicken) may seem small, while other serving sizes (especially for vegetables and fruits) may seem large. All of the portion sizes that I suggest reflect the current Food Guide Pyramid recommendations.

I hope these examples begin to dispel current notions of "portion distortion." As you replace empty-calorie foods with tricklers, fiber, and heart-healthy foods, you'll be amazed at how *so little* (smaller portions and fewer calories) can go *so far* (your energy level). Try not to eat with your eyes, but with your head. A wonderful surprise awaits you!

1,200 daily calories	1,500 daily calories	1,800 daily calories	2,000 daily calories	2,400 daily calories

Ideal calorie range for:

➤ Preadolescent children

➤ Most women who want to lose weight

➤ Inactive adults of small stature

Ideal calorie range for:

➤ Most preteen adolescents

➤ Active women

➤ Older men

➤ Most men who want to lose weight

Ideal calorie range for:

➤ Active teenagers

➤ Large-stature active women

➤ Healthy-weight adult men

Quick-Muffin Breakfast

Fiber-High Bran Muffin*
1 tbs. peanut butter
8 oz. no-sugar-added hot chocolate or 8 oz. skim or 1% milk

Fiber-High Bran Muffin*
1/2 tbs. light margarine
1/2 cup unsweetened canned fruit cocktail
8 oz. no-sugar-added hot chocolate or 8 oz. skim or 1% milk

Fiber-High Bran Muffin*
1 tbs. light cream cheese
Large piece seasonal fruit or 2 cups sliced strawberries
8 oz. no-sugar-added hot chocolate or 8 oz. skim or 1% milk

2 Fiber-High Bran Muffins*
1 tbs. apple butter
1 tbs. light margarine
Large piece seasonal fruit or 2 cups sliced strawberries
8 oz. no-sugar-added hot chocolate or 8 oz. skim or 1% milk

Fiber-High Bran Muffin*
1 tbs. apple butter
2 slices rye or 100% whole wheat toast
2 oz. low-salt boiled ham or reduced-fat cheese
Large piece seasonal fruit or 2 cups sliced strawberries
8 oz. no-sugar-added hot chocolate or 8 oz. skim or 1% milk

*Recipe appears on page 153.

1,200 daily calories	1,500 daily calories	1,800 daily calories	2,000 daily calories	2,400 daily calories
Super Cereal Breakfast				
1⅓ cups Special K	1⅓ cups Special K	1½ cups Special K	2 cups Special K	2 cups Special K
6 oz. skim or 1% milk	8 oz. skim or 1% milk	8 oz. skim or 1% milk	16 oz. skim or 1% milk	16 oz. skim or 1% milk
1 cup unsweetened canned peaches or 1 cup grapes	1 cup unsweetened canned peaches or 1 cup grapes	1 cup unsweetened canned peaches or 1 cup grapes	2 cups unsweetened canned peaches or 2 cups grapes	1 cup unsweetened canned peaches or 1 cup grapes
		Quaker chewy granola bar or 2 low-fat graham crackers (2 full sheets)	Quaker chewy granola bar or 2 low-fat graham crackers (2 full sheets)	2 Quaker chewy granola bars or 4 low-fat graham crackers (4 full sheets)
Cooked Cereal Breakfast				
½ cup dry old-fashioned oats cooked with water	½ cup dry old-fashioned oats cooked with water	½ cup dry old-fashioned oats cooked with 1 cup skim or 1% milk	½ cup dry old-fashioned oats cooked with 1 cup skim or 1% milk	¾ cup dry old-fashioned oats cooked with 1½ cups skim or 1% milk
½ cup Simply Delicious Applesauce* or 1 cup unsweetened canned peaches	½ cup Simply Delicious Applesauce* or 1 cup unsweetened canned peaches	½ cup Simply Delicious Applesauce* or 1 cup unsweetened canned peaches	½ cup Simply Delicious Applesauce* or 1 cup unsweetened canned peaches	½ cup Simply Delicious Applesauce* or 1 cup unsweetened canned peaches
	4 oz. light yogurt	1 low-fat graham cracker (1 full sheet)	1 sourdough or whole wheat English muffin	1 sourdough or whole-wheat English muffin
			1 tbs. natural, no-salt-added peanut butter	2 tsp. natural, no-salt-added peanut butter
			2 tsp. all-fruit spread	2 tsp. all-fruit spread

*Recipe appears on page 202.

1,200 daily calories	1,500 daily calories	1,800 daily calories	2,000 daily calories	2,400 daily calories
Delicious Deli Lunch				
2 slices rye bread	2 slices rye bread	2 slices rye bread	2 slices rye bread	2 slices rye bread
1 oz. turkey breast	1 oz. turkey breast	1 oz. turkey breast	2 oz. turkey breast	2 oz. turkey breast
1 oz. low-fat cheese	1 oz. low-fat cheese	1 oz. low-fat cheese	2 oz. low-fat cheese	2 oz. low-fat cheese
Lettuce	Lettuce	Lettuce	Lettuce	Lettuce
Tomato	Tomato	Tomato	Tomato	Tomato
1 cup cantaloupe or 1 orange	1 cup cantaloupe or 1 orange	1 cup cantaloupe or 1 orange	1½ cups cantaloupe or 1 medium apple	1 tbs. light mayonnaise
4 oz. light yogurt	8 oz. light yogurt	8 oz. light yogurt	8 oz. light yogurt	2 cups cantaloupe or 2 cups grapes
				8 oz. light yogurt
				4 Fifty 50 vanilla wafers
Wrap Lunch				
Goat Cheese Wrap*	Goat Cheese Wrap*	Goat Cheese Wrap*	Goat Cheese Wrap*	2 Goat Cheese Wraps*
1 cup lettuce, tomato, cucumber, and red onion salad	1 cup lettuce, tomato, cucumber, and red onion salad	1 cup lettuce, tomato, cucumber, and red onion salad	1 cup lettuce, tomato, cucumber, and red onion salad	1 cup lettuce, tomato, cucumber, and red onion salad
2 tbs. Good Seasons fat-free dressing	2 tbs. Good Seasons fat-free dressing	2 tbs. Good Seasons fat-free dressing	2 tbs. Good Seasons fat-free dressing	2 tbs. Good Seasons fat-free dressing
4 Pringles Right crisps (⅓ less fat)	8 Pringles Right crisps (⅓ less fat)	8 Pringles Right crisps (⅓ less fat)	8 Pringles Right crisps (⅓ less fat)	1 kiwi or 1 cup strawberries
			2 kiwis or 2 cups strawberries	

*Recipe appears on page 192.

1,200 daily calories	1,500 daily calories	1,800 daily calories	2,000 daily calories	2,400 daily calories

Salad Bar Lunch

1,200 daily calories	1,500 daily calories	1,800 daily calories	2,000 daily calories	2,400 daily calories
1 cup lettuce	1 cup lettuce	1 cup lettuce	1 cup lettuce	1 cup lettuce
2 cups mixed raw vegetables	2 cups mixed raw vegetables	2 cups mixed raw vegetables	2 cups mixed raw vegetables	2 cups mixed raw vegetables
½ cup kidney beans	½ cup kidney beans	½ cup kidney beans	½ cup kidney beans	½ cup kidney beans
¼ cup reduced-fat salad dressing	¼ cup reduced-fat salad dressing	¼ cup reduced-fat salad dressing	¼ cup reduced-fat salad dressing	1 hard-boiled egg
2 Ry-Krisp crackers	3 Ry-Krisp crackers	3 Ry-Krisp crackers	3 Ry-Krisp crackers	¼ cup reduced-fat salad dressing
2 Fifty 50 oatmeal cookies	3 Fifty 50 oatmeal cookies	3 Fifty 50 oatmeal cookies	3 Fifty 50 oatmeal cookies	3 Ry-Krisp crackers
			1 medium pear or 8 oz. canned unsweetened pears	6 Fifty 50 oatmeal cookies
				1 medium pear or 8 oz. canned, unsweetened pears

Pasta Dinner

1,200 daily calories	1,500 daily calories	1,800 daily calories	2,000 daily calories	2,400 daily calories
1 cup Just-Plain-Good Pasta*	1½ cup Just-Plain-Good Pasta*	1½ cup Just-Plain-Good Pasta*	1½ cup Just-Plain-Good Pasta*	2 cups Just-Plain-Good Pasta*
3 oz. chicken breast, skinless, grilled	3 oz. chicken breast, skinless, grilled	3 oz. chicken breast, skinless, grilled	6 oz. chicken breast, skinless, grilled	6 oz. chicken breast, skinless, grilled
6 asparagus spears, steamed or grilled	9 asparagus spears, steamed or grilled	9 asparagus spears, steamed or grilled	9 asparagus spears, steamed or grilled	12 asparagus spears, steamed or grilled
1 tsp. olive oil or ½ tbs. light whipped margarine	1 tsp. olive oil or ½ tbs. light whipped margarine	1 tsp. olive oil or ½ tbs. light whipped margarine	1 tsp. olive oil or ½ tbs. light whipped margarine	1 tsp. olive oil or ½ tbs. light whipped margarine
½ cup cooked, sugar-free pudding	½ cup cooked, sugar-free pudding	½ cup cooked, sugar-free pudding	Small baked apple or 1 cup sliced strawberries	Small baked apple or 1 cup sliced strawberries
1 tbs. Cool Whip Lite or Dream Whip	1 tbs. Cool Whip Lite or Dream Whip	1 tbs. Cool Whip Lite or Dream Whip	1 tbs. whipped topping	1 tbs. whipped topping

*Recipe appears on page 182.

1,200 daily calories	1,500 daily calories	1,800 daily calories	2,000 daily calories	2,400 daily calories
Fish Dinner				
½ cup Saffron Rice Pilaf*	¾ cup Saffron Rice Pilaf*	¾ cup Saffron Rice Pilaf*	1 cup Saffron Rice Pilaf*	1 cup Saffron Rice Pilaf*
3 oz. wild salmon, grilled or poached, or 6 oz. cod, broiled	4 oz. wild salmon, grilled or poached, or 8 oz. cod, broiled	4 oz. wild salmon, grilled or poached, or 8 oz. cod, broiled	4 oz. wild salmon, grilled or poached, or 8 oz. cod, broiled	5 oz. wild salmon, grilled or poached, or 10 oz. cod, broiled
1½ cups or 2 stalks broccoli, steamed	1 cup or 1 stalk broccoli, steamed	1 cup or 1 stalk broccoli, steamed	1 cup or 1 stalk broccoli, steamed	1½ cups or 2 stalks broccoli, steamed
2 tsp. olive oil or 1 tbs. light whipped margarine	2 tsp. olive oil or 1 tbs. light whipped margarine	2 tsp. olive oil or 1 tbs. light whipped margarine	2 tsp. olive oil or 1 tbs. light whipped margarine	2 tsp. olive oil or 1 tbs. light whipped margarine
1 cup citrus sections or 1½ cups fresh fruit salad	1 cup citrus sections or 1½ cups fresh fruit salad	1 cup citrus sections or 1½ cups fresh fruit salad	1 cup citrus sections or 1½ cups fresh fruit salad	1 cup citrus sections or 1½ cups fresh fruit salad

*Recipe appears on page 168

1,200 daily calories	1,500 daily calories	1,800 daily calories	2,000 daily calories	2,400 daily calories
Meatless Dinner				
1 cup So-Sweet Pepper Soup*	1 cup So-Sweet Pepper Soup*	1 cup So-Sweet Pepper Soup*	1½ cups So-Sweet Pepper Soup*	1½ cups So-Sweet Pepper Soup*
2-egg mushroom omelet	2-egg mushroom omelet	2-egg mushroom omelet	2-egg mushroom omelet	2-egg and 1-oz. low-fat cheddar-mushroom omelet
Mini-pita, toasted	2-oz. pita, toasted	2-oz. pita, toasted	2-oz. pita, toasted	2-oz. pita, toasted
1 cup steamed green beans or spinach	1 cup steamed green beans or spinach	1 cup steamed green beans or spinach	1 cup steamed green beans or spinach	2 cups steamed green beans or spinach
1 tsp. olive oil	1 tsp. olive oil	1 tsp. olive oil	2 tsp. olive oil	2 tsp. olive oil
2 fresh apricots or ¾ cup sliced strawberries	4 fresh apricots or 1½ cups sliced strawberries	4 fresh apricots or 1½ cups sliced strawberries	4 fresh apricots or 1½ cups sliced strawberries	4 fresh apricots or 1½ cups sliced strawberries

*Recipe appears on page 160.

The Snack Shack

Here is a list of snack calories for every calorie plan below. No matter which meal plan you choose, it's okay to eat snacks. In fact, it's one of my preferred strategies that I offer to my patients to help them feel energetic and satisfied throughout the day. So, for example, for a 1,200-calorie day, add in 100 snack calories. And if your meal plan calls for a 200-calorie snack, you can choose two 100-calorie snacks or one 200-calorie snack, and so on.

1,200 daily calories: Add in 100 snack calories
1,500 daily calories: Add in 200 snack calories
1,800 daily calories: Add in 400 snack calories
2,000 daily calories: Add in 200 snack calories
2,400 daily calories: Add in 300 snack calories

Here are some trickler snacks that will keep you feeling satisfied no matter how many calories you're eating.

100-Calorie Snacks

- 1 Quaker chewy granola bar
- 3 Fifty 50 oatmeal cookies
- 4 sections Fifty 50 sugar-free milk chocolate
- 11 sourdough pretzel nuggets
- 28 pistachios
- 8 walnut halves
- 22 dry-roasted peanuts
- 29 cherries
- 1¼ cups blueberries
- 1¾ cups grapes (about 30 large grapes)
- 8 oz. skim or 1% milk
- 6–8 oz. light yogurt
- 1 pear
- 1½ cups honeydew
- 17 small baked tortilla chips and ¼ cup refrigerated salsa
- ½ cup soft-serve frozen yogurt

⟩ ½ cup ice milk

⟩ ⅛ slice avocado and 3 Ry-Krisp crackers

⟩ 1 oz. part-skim mozzarella and 1 Wasa bread

200-Calorie Snacks

⟩ 1 Fiber-High Bran Muffin[1] and 1 tbs. all-fruit jelly

⟩ 6 Lorna Doone cookies

⟩ ¼ cup soy nuts

⟩ 26 dry-roasted almonds

⟩ 1 cup Simply Delicious Applesauce[2]

⟩ 7 dried peach halves

⟩ ¾ cup Healthy Choice ice cream

⟩ 6 to 8 oz. light yogurt and ¼ cup High-Test Granola[3]

⟩ 12 oz. skim or 1% milk and 2 tbs. Lite Hershey chocolate syrup

⟩ 6 stoneground wheat crackers and 2 tbs. hummus

⟩ 1 fruit smoothie (8 oz. skim or 1% milk and 1½–2 cups frozen berries)

⟩ 1 Pizzetta[4]

⟩ 1 Chocolate Applesauce Cupcake[5]

---

[1] *Recipe appears on page 153*

[2] *Recipe appears on page 202*

[3] *Recipe appears on page 152*

[4] *Recipe appears on page 196*

[5] *Recipe appears on page 199*

To Wrap Up

We all know from our own experiences that doing the *same* things in the *same* ways will produce the *same* results. If you are not willing to keep your current health and energy levels status quo, then, are you ready to try something *different*? This is the question I pose to my patients who come to see me in my office, and this is the same question I pose to my virtual patients, the readers of this book. I give my office patients the facts—not my opinion—about how the body works and how food works in the body. I listen to their specific health concerns; I answer their questions with my best nutritional wisdom. I encourage them to make the choices that make the most sense to them, which they then make on their terms.

In this book I have written down the overlapping contents of the daily conversations that I have been having with my patients for nearly twenty years. If the reader interacts with the information I've presented in this book, there is not a doubt in my mind that the same positive lifestyle changes that I see in my office will ensue "out there."

THE BOTTOM LINE

A Great Carb Is . . .

- ➤ Whole, not refined or enriched
- ➤ High in fiber and nutrient-dense
- ➤ Dense, not airy or puffed
- ➤ Unprocessed, or minimally processed
- ➤ Natural

A Great Diet Is . . .

- ➤ Balanced: great carbs (55 to 60 percent), high quality proteins (10 to 15 percent) and heart healthy fats (30 percent)
- ➤ Wholesome
- ➤ Good for your health
- ➤ Not a diet! It's a lifestyle

PART 3

Recipes

About These Recipes
(please read)

I would like to give my readers the same recipe ideas I offer to my patients, so here are a few of the most popular ones. Because I lived in Italy for many years, I frequently draw from my Italian cooking experiences. You will surely note that influence in my recipes.

Since this is a book primarily about carbohydrates, I'm only presenting carbohydrate-rich recipes. Some are main dishes while others are soups, salads, or side dishes of grains or vegetables. And then there are some breakfast and snack ideas, too. I hope you will choose a few each month and make them your own.

You may notice that a few of these recipes may seem high in fat. This is because, in these particular recipes, there is a considerable amount of whole-grain flour (which contains the natural oils from the bran layer), or nuts, or oils or margarines that are considered heart-healthy (those that contain no trans fats). While these remain healthful recipes, if you are watching your calories, you can eat a smaller portion of these foods or combine them with lower-fat foods in the meal. This is the recommendation I give to my patients and one, of course, that I adhere to myself. Having said this, I divided each recipe into what I would consider an appropriate serving size for that food when used as indicated (for example, I am suggesting that you eat 1½ cups of the tortellini and ham salad as your *main dish not as a side dish*).

In addition to the nutritional analysis, I also have listed for each recipe the glycemic index value and the glycemic load for the recommended serving size. You will see LOW, MODERATE, or HIGH. Take a look at these values. They drive home the idea of nutrient density as well as serving as a reminder that we should not choose a food solely on its GI or GL values but rather adjust portion sizes (up or down) based on these qualities.

Sure, you could purchase some of these dishes and just heat and serve them. But, in my opinion, no commercially prepared food could ever match up to your good, wholesome cooking! If your time is at a premium, make extra food for the next day or freeze it (at least you'll know what's in that frozen package). If you're on a tight budget, buy fresh foods in season and staples in bulk or on sale. Read through each recipe carefully *before* executing it so there is no waste of time or ingredients.

Finally, it is my hope that you will enjoy preparing these foods and that you will allow your body to acknowledge and receive the nourishment of each ingredient you feed it. I'd like to remind you to be present to the process of taking care of your body by offering it wholesome foods, prepared by you with the mindful addition of the most important ingredients of all, appreciation and respect for your body and the foods that nourish it.

BREAKFAST FOODS

Breakfast Pockets

BREAKFAST is the most important meal of the day. This simple egg-filled pita is loaded with nutrients and long-lasting energy. Can you think of a better way to say "Good morning" to your body?

〖 **Makes 2 servings   Serving size: 2 pocket halves** 〗

2 strips	center-cut bacon[1]
2	scallions, green part only
1	egg[2]
¾ cup	egg substitute
Pinch	salt
Pinch	pepper, freshly ground
	cooking spray
2 2-oz.	whole wheat pitas (with pockets)
4 tbs.	salsa[3]

1. Place the bacon strips in a preheated, nonstick skillet and cook over medium-high heat, about one minute on each side (be careful of splattering). When done, remove the strips from the skillet and drain on paper towels. When cooled, crumble the bacon into a small dish and set aside.
2. Clean the skillet with paper towels and set aside.
3. Wash and pat dry the scallions. Cut them into thin horizontal slices. Place in small dish and set aside.
4. In a small mixing bowl, whisk together the egg and egg substitute, and a pinch each of salt and freshly ground pepper.
5. Spray and preheat the skillet (avoid burning). Add the egg mixture, stirring frequently, especially around the edges, until scrambled, approximately 3 minutes.
6. Remove the eggs to a separate dish and keep warm.
7. Reduce heat to low and warm each pita on both sides in the skillet, then cut them in half.

8. Divide the eggs, bacon, and scallions in fourths. Fill each pita pocket in this order: (1) eggs, (2) bacon, (3) scallions.

9. Top each pocket with a tablespoon of salsa. Serve immediately.

EACH SERVING CONTAINS:
206 calories, 22 grams carbohydrates, 18 grams protein, 5 grams fat, 98 milligrams cholesterol, 3 grams fiber

GI = LOW   GL = MODERATE

[1] Other lean choices are Canadian bacon or vegetable protein breakfast strips.

[2] I use eggs from cage-free hens.

[3] Try a fruit-based salsa, like peach and chipotle, with no preservatives.

High-Test Granola

MAKE this recipe just once, taste it just once, and store-bought granola will be wiped off your shopping list forever!

〖 Makes 9 cups Serving size: ½ cup 〗

	vegetable spray
½ cup	honey
6 cups	old-fashioned oats (not quick oats)
1 tbs.	cinnamon
¼ cup	ground flaxseed
¾ cup	slivered almonds (or any other nut, such as pecans, cashews, almonds, or walnuts), toasted
¼ cup	soy nuts
1 cup	dried blueberries and currants (or any other combination of dried fruit, except dates)

1. Spray a large baking pan (9″ × 10″ × 2½″) with cooking spray. Add the honey.
2. Place the pan in cold oven. Turn on oven to 350°.
3. In a large bowl, combine the next 5 ingredients (oats through soy nuts). Mix well.
4. When the honey has melted, remove the pan from oven. Add the oat mixture to the baking pan. Spread and turn to coat well with honey.
5. Bake for 25 minutes or until the oats are well toasted, turning every 5 to 6 minutes.
6. Remove from the oven. Cool thoroughly.
7. Add the dried fruit.
8. Store in airtight container.

EACH SERVING CONTAINS:
200 calories, 31 grams carbohydrate, 7 grams protein, 5 grams fat, 0 milligrams cholesterol, 5 grams fiber

GI = LOW   GL = MODERATE

Fiber-High Bran Muffins

THESE small muffins certainly pack a powerful energy punch. Top with a little dab of peanut butter and you're ready for several hours on the fast track.

❨ **Makes 48 muffins   Serving: 1 muffin** ❩

2 cups	boiling water
5 tsp.	baking soda
1 quart	low-fat buttermilk
¾ cup	margarine, room temperature
2 cups	sugar
2	eggs
½ cup	egg substitute
2 cups	bran flakes
4 cups	All-Bran with Extra Fiber
5 cups	whole wheat flour
1 cup	walnuts, coarsely chopped
1 cup	dried blueberries (or 2 cups fresh), optional

1. Preheat oven to 425°. Spray 4 muffin tins with vegetable spray.
2. Pour the boiling water into a medium-sized bowl, add the baking soda, then the buttermilk. Let cool.
3. Place the margarine, sugar, eggs, and egg substitute in a medium bowl. Beat for 2 minutes at medium speed until smooth.
4. Place both cereals in a food processor fitted with a steel blade. Process until coarsely ground.
5. Pour cereals into a large mixing bowl. Add in the flour.
6. Alternately add the buttermilk and creamed margarine mixture to the dry ingredients.
7. Fold in the walnuts and fruit, if adding.
8. Bake 20 minutes.

154

EACH SERVING CONTAINS:
141 calories, 24 grams carbohydrate, 3 grams protein, 5 grams fat, 10 milligrams cholesterol, 4 grams fiber

GI = LOW   GL = MODERATE

Apple'n'Oats
Breakfast Pudding

HERE is a fabulous invitation to a great day! When you taste the combination of these flavors you'll know they were made for each other.

2 cups	skim milk
1 tbs.	tub margarine or light butter
¼ tsp.	cinnamon
⅛ tsp	salt
3 tbs.	brown sugar
1	medium apple (peeled, cored, and diced)[1]
1 cup	rolled oats
1 tsp.	vanilla
¼ tsp.	nutmeg
	cooking spray

1. Preheat the oven to 350°.
2. Spray a 1-quart baking dish with cooking spray.
3. Combine the first 5 ingredients (milk through brown sugar) in a 2-quart saucepan. Heat on high for 4 minutes to scald the milk.
4. Add the apple pieces and the oats. Continue cooking on high for 1 minute. Remove from heat and stir in the vanilla.
5. Pour the mixture into the prepared baking dish. Bake for 15 minutes.
6. Remove from the oven. Stir the mixture thoroughly. Sprinkle the top with nutmeg. Return to oven and bake for 15 minutes.
7. Serve warm with 1 tablespoon cream, if desired.

156

EACH SERVING CONTAINS:
166 calories, 27 grams carbohydrates, 8 grams protein, 3 grams fat, 0 milligrams cholesterol, 3 grams fiber

GI = LOW **GL = MODERATE**
[1] Good baking apples are Macintosh, Cortland, Jonathan, Winesap, Rome Beauty.

30-Second
Breakfast Eggnog

THIS recipe eliminates your "I-have-no-time" excuse for skipping breakfast. And come mid-morning, you'll be delighted with the energy your body will still be receiving from this delicious drink.

⟨ **Makes 2 servings   Serving size: 10 oz** ⟩

4 oz.	vanilla or raspberry light yogurt
4 oz.	nonfat milk
1 cup	raspberries, fresh or frozen
½ cup	egg substitute
2 tbs.	cocoa powder
1 tbs.	honey

Combine all ingredients in a blender. Mix at high speed for 30 seconds until smooth. Serve immediately.

EACH SERVING CONTAINS:
160 calories, 28 grams carbohydrate; 12 grams protein, 2 grams fat; 0 milligrams cholesterol, 6 grams fiber

GI = LOW   **GL = LOW**

Soups

So-Sweet Pepper Soup

WHO would have thought that this humble combination of vegetables would produce such a hardy-tasting soup?

〖 Makes 9 cups   Serving size: 1½ cups 〗

1 tbs.	olive oil
1	medium onion, coarsely chopped
1½	large celery stalks, coarsely chopped
2 cloves	garlic, minced
4 cups	low-sodium vegetable stock
2 cups	water
1½ cup (8 oz.)	creamer potatoes,[1] cubed
5	yellow bell peppers, halved, seeded, and quartered
½ tsp.	salt
⅛ tsp.	freshly ground pepper
3 cups	boiling water
1 cup	barley, uncooked

Homemade or commercial pesto sauce, to garnish (optional)
Grated Reggiano Parmesan cheese, to garnish (optional)

1. In a large, wide-based saucepan, heat the oil over medium-low heat. Add the onions and celery; sauté 4 minutes. Add the garlic and continue to sauté another 3 minutes (onions will be soft and translucent).
2. Add the next six ingredients (vegetable stock through ground pepper); bring to a boil. Reduce heat, cover, and simmer for 40 to 45 minutes.
3. While the vegetables are cooking, in a separate medium saucepan bring 3 cups of water to a boil and add the barley.
4. Reduce heat, cover, and simmer for 30 minutes; add more water if needed. Stir occasionally.
5. When cooked, drain the barley and reserve in a large saucepan.
6. When the vegetables are cooked, pour half of the mixture into a blender and process until completely

smooth. Pour the pureed mixture into pan with the barley. Heat on low to keep warm.

7. Repeat with the remaining pepper mixture. Stir thoroughly.

8. Garnish with a dime-size dollop of pesto and grated cheese if desired.

EACH SERVING CONTAINS:
174 calories, 36 grams carbohydrate, 5 grams protein, 3 grams fat, 0 milligrams cholesterol, 6 grams fiber

GI = LOW   GL= LOW

[1] Creamer potatoes are whole new potatoes with a thin, yellowish skin.

Pasta with Beans

SOUPS are a great way to enjoy a variety of flavors and nutrients with minimal preparation. This soup is no exception—and you'll have leftovers for the next day!

{ **Makes 14 cups   Serving size: 2 cups** }

1 15½-oz. can	light red kidney beans
1 large	celery stalk, preferably with leaves, sliced into 8–10 pieces
2	canned whole plum tomatoes, quartered
1 small	onion, thickly sliced
1 clove	garlic, coarsely chopped
6 large leaves	fresh basil, hand-ripped into quarters
3 sprigs	fresh parsley, leaves only
2 quarts (8 cups)	vegetable or chicken broth
1½ cups	uncooked small pasta (shells, elbows, ditalini)
	salt and pepper, to taste

1. Rinse and drain the beans. Place them in a 4-quart saucepan.
2. Place the next 6 ingredients (celery through parsley) in a food processor. Pulse 8 to 10 times. Add to the beans and stir through.
3. Add the broth and bring to boil.
4. Reduce to low-moderate heat, cover and cook for 15 minutes, stirring occasionally.
5. Add the pasta, mix thoroughly. Cook uncovered for 10 minutes or until the pasta is cooked. Stir occasionally.
6. Correct seasoning to taste. Serve piping hot or warm.

EACH SERVING CONTAINS:
162 calories, 32 grams carbohydrate; 7 grams protein, less than 1 gram fat, 0 milligrams cholesterol, 4 grams fiber

GI = LOW   GL = LOW

Chicken Barley Soup

THIS is a lot of good nutrition in just one bowl. Make extra and freeze it for when you have the sniffles or just want a comfort food on a wintry day.

(Makes 6 servings   Serving size: 1½ cups)

1 lb.	skinless chicken breast
½ cup	pearl barley
1 tbs.	extra-virgin olive oil
1½ cups	carrots, thinly sliced (about 3 medium)
1½ cups	celery, thinly sliced (about 3 stalks including leaves)
1	small onion, chopped
2 cups	sliced mushrooms (about 4 oz.)
½ bunch	fresh spinach, stems removed (about 4 cups)
1 15½-oz. can	diced tomatoes
	salt and pepper to taste

1. Pour 4 cups of cold water into a 2-quart saucepan. Add the chicken. Bring to a boil, removing any scum that forms. Reduce the heat, cover and poach for 25 minutes.
2. In the meantime, bring 2 cups of water to a boil in a 3-quart saucepan. Add the barley, cover and simmer for 40 minutes, stirring occasionally.
3. Pour a tablespoon of the olive oil in a large skillet. Add the carrots, celery, and onion. Sauté 3 minutes. Add the mushrooms and sauté for an additional 3 minutes.
4. Remove the vegetables from the heat and add the barley when cooked.
5. Remove the chicken from the poaching broth and cube. Pour the broth into the barley and vegetables. Add in the chicken.
6. Add the spinach and the tomatoes, with their juice, to the soup. Bring to a boil, cover and simmer for 10 minutes. Before serving, correct for seasoning.

164

EACH SERVING CONTAINS:
178 calories, 19 grams carbohydrate; 18 grams
protein, 4 grams fat, 35 milligrams cholesterol,
5 grams fiber

GI = LOW   GL = LOW

Mom's "Kicked Up" Lentil Soup

THE B vitamins, potassium, iron and phosphorus in the lentils combined with the antioxidants in the red wine make a cup of this soup a healthy fill-up! And just one serving provides more than 50 percent of an adult's daily fiber requirement.

❨ **Makes 8 cups   Serving size: 1½ cups** ❩

5 cups	beef or vegetable broth
1 cup	brown lentils, rinsed
6	medium carrots, thinly sliced
2	celery stalks, including leaves, thinly sliced
1	large onion, coarsely chopped
1	bay leaf
1 cup	dry red wine
	pepper, freshly ground
	grated Parmesan cheese, optional

1. Combine the first 6 ingredients (broth through bay leaf) in a large saucepan or stock pot. Bring to a boil, cover and simmer for 45 minutes.
2. Add the wine and freshly ground pepper to taste. Cook over medium heat for 5 minutes.
3. Serve hot with a sprinkle of grated cheese if desired.

EACH SERVING CONTAINS:
202 calories, 37 grams carbohydrate, 10 grams protein, 0 grams fat, 0 milligrams cholesterol, 14 grams fiber

GI = LOW   GL = MODERATE

SIDE DISHES AND SALADS

168

Saffron Rice Pilaf

THIS colorful rice dish blends flavorful ingredients into a definite crowd-pleaser.

(**Makes 4 cups   Serving size: ½ cup**)

½ tbs.	olive oil
1 small	onion, finely chopped
2 cloves	garlic, minced
1 cup	Uncle Ben's Converted Rice
Dash	saffron threads
2½ cups	hot broth (chicken or vegetable)
1 tsp.	salt (omit if broth is not low sodium)
2 tbs.	fresh parsley (4 sprigs), finely chopped

1. Heat the oil in a medium saucepan over medium heat. Add the onion and sauté until soft, about 4 to 5 minutes.
2. Add the garlic and sauté for another 2 minutes (do not let garlic turn brown).
3. Add the rice and saffron and stir to coat with the oil.
4. Add the hot broth and salt (if used) and stir gently. Reduce heat and cover.
5. Simmer for 20 minutes.
6. Remove from heat; let rest for 5 minutes.
7. Add the parsley. Fluff the rice with fork and serve.

EACH SERVING CONTAINS:
97 calories, 20 grams carbohydrate, 2 grams protein, 1 gram fat, 0 milligrams cholesterol, 2 grams fiber

GI = LOW   GL = LOW

Smashed
Sweet Potato-Carrot
Puree

DON'T save this recipe just for Thanksgiving dinner. Why not give your body the vitamin A, potassium, and fiber contained in both the sweet potatoes and carrots throughout the year—and delight your taste buds at the same time?

⟨ **Makes 4½ cups   Serving size: ½ cup** ⟩

2 lbs.	sweet potatoes or yams, scrubbed, ends cut off
1 lb.	baby carrots
2 cups	water
1 tbs.	brown sugar
3 tbs.	butter or margarine
	salt and pepper to taste
½ cup	light sour cream
½ tsp.	nutmeg
1 tbs.	cognac or port or sherry wine

1. Bake, steam, or microwave the sweet potatoes until tender. (Time will depend on size of potato and cooking method; the longest cooking time: baked for one hour at 375°.)
2. Place the carrots in medium saucepan with 2 cups water, the brown sugar, butter or margarine, salt, and pepper. Cook, uncovered, over medium heat about 30 minutes or until tender, making sure all water has evaporated. When cooked, place in the bowl of a food processor fitted with a steel blade.
3. When sweet potatoes are cooked, cool for easy handling. Scrape out the flesh with a spoon and add potatoes to carrots in the processor.
4. Combine the sour cream, nutmeg, and cognac or wine. Add to the vegetables and process until very smooth.
5. Taste to correct seasonings.

6. Transfer the puree to a 9-inch-square baking dish, cover, and heat thoroughly in an oven preheated to 350°.

7. Serve steaming hot.

> **EACH SERVING CONTAINS:**
> 130 calories, 20 grams carbohydrate, 2 grams protein, 5 grams fat, 14 milligrams cholesterol, 3 grams fiber

GI = LOW   GL = LOW

Old World Vegetable Stew

THIS versatile mixture of vegetables and herbs will enhance the flavors of rice, pasta, couscous, or pita bread. It mixes so well with so many staples, it can easily become a staple itself!

(**Makes 10 servings   Serving size: 1 cup**)

2 tbs.	olive oil
1	large garlic clove, minced
2 medium	onions, thickly sliced
1 medium	eggplant (approx. 12 oz.), unpeeled and cubed
1 medium	red bell pepper, seeded and sliced into 2-inch strips
1 medium	green bell pepper, seeded and sliced into 2-inch strips
2 large	yellow or green squash, thickly sliced
4 medium	tomatoes, peeled and seeded, cut into eighths (or 1 20-oz. can of plum tomatoes, drained, seeded, and quartered)
1 12-oz.	jar marinated artichoke hearts, drained and quartered
1 tbs.	fresh thyme, or ½ tsp. dried
1 tbs.	fresh oregano, or ½ tsp. dried
2 tbs.	fresh basil, minced, or ½ tsp. dried
⅛ cup	balsamic vinegar
½ tsp.	freshly ground black pepper
2 tbs.	fresh parsley, finely chopped

1. Heat the oil in large saucepan. Add the garlic and onions, and cook over low heat until onions are soft.
2. Add the eggplant, peppers, and squash and continue to cook over medium heat for 5 minutes, stirring frequently.
3. Add the tomatoes, artichoke hearts, and herbs and mix well. Cover and simmer for 20 minutes, stirring frequently.
4. Stir in the balsamic vinegar. Continue to cook, uncovered, for 5 minutes, stirring frequently.

5. Add the black pepper and parsley; mix thoroughly. May be served hot or at room temperature.

> **EACH SERVING CONTAINS:**
> 101 calories, 15 grams carbohydrate, 1 gram protein, 6 grams fat, 4 grams fiber, 0 milligrams cholesterol

GI = LOW   GL = LOW

Mashed Cauliflower

IT'S not what you think it is (mashed potatoes) but tastes at least as good. Watch the kids lap up this veggie and ask for seconds!

❮ **Makes 2½ cups   Serving size: ½ cup** ❯

1	medium-head cauliflower (approx. 6 cups)
1 tbs.	tub margarine or light butter
¾ cup	leeks, thinly sliced horizontally
1 clove	garlic, minced
	salt
1–2 tbs.	grated Parmesan cheese

1. Remove the outer leaves of the cauliflower. Break or cut the head into small florets. Wash and place in a vegetable steamer in a saucepan with 1″ of water.
2. Cook over medium-high heat for 10 to 15 minutes, until tender. Cooking time will depend on the size of the florets.
3. While the cauliflower is steaming, melt the margarine in a small skillet. Sauté the leeks for 3 minutes. When they start browning, add the garlic and sauté another minute. Remove from heat. Salt to taste.
4. Place all the vegetables in a food processor. Process at high speed for about 45 seconds until a smooth puree results.
5. Transfer to a serving dish. Sprinkle with cheese. Serve hot.

EACH SERVING CONTAINS:
70 calories, 11 grams carbohydrate, 4 grams protein, 2 grams fat, 1 milligram cholesterol, 6 grams fiber

GI = LOW   GL = LOW

Marinated Eggplant Slices with Herbs

THIS recipe can be made on the spot or in advance of a meal. You can also use one or two of these eggplant slices to slip inside a sandwich to enhance both flavor and daily vegetable consumption!

【 Makes 15 slices   Serving size: 3 slices 】

1	eggplant (1¼ lbs.)
2 tbs.	coarse salt
	cooking spray
1 cup	canned tomatoes, diced
1 large clove	garlic, minced
¼ cup	red onion, diced
½ cup	loose thyme leaves (about 15 sprigs)
1 tbs.	extra-virgin olive oil
1 tbs.	lemon juice, freshly squeezed

1. Remove the stem end of the eggplant. Cut it into 15 round slices.
2. Fill a large bowl three-quarters full with water. Add the salt and the eggplant slices. Let them soak for at least 20 minutes to remove bitterness.
3. Turn on the broiler to high. Coat a baking sheet with cooking spray.
4. Remove the eggplant slices from the salted water. Pat them dry with paper towels and spread them in a single layer on the baking sheet.
5. Broil 4½" from the heat for a total of 8 minutes, 5 minutes on the first side, and 3 minutes when turned over. Remove from the oven and arrange the slices slightly overlapping each other on large platter.
6. Mix the next 6 ingredients (tomatoes through lemon juice) in a small mixing bowl.
7. Distribute the tomato-herb mixture evenly over the eggplant. Cover and let stand for several hours at room temperature before serving. You can also refrigerate

overnight—just bring the dish to room temperature before serving.

EACH SERVING CONTAINS:
60 calories, 7 grams carbohydrate, 1 gram protein,
3 grams fat, 0 milligrams cholesterol, 3 grams fiber

GI = LOW   GL = LOW

Herbed Balsamic Mushrooms

EVEN though mushrooms are 90 percent water, they contain fiber, are rich in potassium and a good source of vitamin B2. This recipe harmoniously combines the natural earthy flavors of the mushrooms and the herbs.

《 **Makes 2 cups - Serving size: ⅔ cup** 》

1 lb.	small portobello mushrooms[1] (approx. 24)
	cooking spray
½ tbs.	olive oil
1 clove	garlic, minced
1 tbs.	fresh rosemary, finely chopped (1–2 sprigs)
½ to 1 tbs.	balsamic vinegar[2]
1 tbs.	fresh parsley, finely chopped (2–3 sprigs)

1. Preheat oven to 450° F.
2. With a mushroom brush or damp cloth, clean tops and bottoms of the mushrooms. Do not wash under running faucet or submerge in water.
3. Lightly cover a jelly-roll pan with cooking spray. Place the mushrooms upside down on the pan.
4. Mix the next 3 ingredients (olive oil through rosemary) in small condiment dish. Brush the mushrooms with the oil mixture and bake for 25 minutes.
4. When done, remove the mushrooms from the oven and slice them and place in serving bowl. Add the vinegar and parsley; toss and serve.

EACH SERVING CONTAINS:
61 calories, 7 grams carbohydrate, 3 grams protein,
3 grams fat, 0 milligrams cholesterol, 2 grams fiber

GL = LOW   GL = LOW

[1] I use the *baby bella* or small portobello mushrooms because they are less expensive than the large ones, more robust, and easier to wash.

[2] How much you use depends on the quality of your balsamic vinegar. The more expensive the vinegar, the denser it is, so use less than a thinner product.

178

White Bean Salad

SIMPLE and quick—this salad has all the markings of convenience. And such nutritious ingredients guarantee a supply of fiber, minerals like potassium, iron, magnesium and copper, and vitamins A, C, B_1, folic acid, and niacin.

❨ **Makes 6 cups   Serving size: ½ cup** ❩

1 19-oz. can	cannellini beans, drained and rinsed
1 14½-oz. can	diced tomatoes[1], drained
1 clove	garlic, minced
½ cup	red onion, chopped
1 tbs.	extra-virgin olive oil
½ tbs.	balsamic vinegar
2 tbs.	fresh parsley, finely chopped (5 sprigs)
¼ tsp.	salt
	freshly ground pepper, to taste
1 oz.	crumbled blue cheese[2]

Combine all ingredients in a medium serving dish. Serve at room temperature.

EACH SERVING CONTAINS:
125 calories, 17 grams carbohydrate, 5 grams protein, 4 grams fat, 4 milligrams cholesterol, 5 grams fiber

GI = LOW   GL = LOW
[1] May substitute with 3 fresh plum tomatoes when in season.
[2] May substitute feta or gorgonzola cheese, if preferred.

Main Dishes

Spaghetti Estate

SURPRISE! Here's a refreshing salad that serves as a "sauce" for spaghetti. This recipe is adapted from a small trattoria in the heart of Rome, famous for its "Summer Spaghetti."

〚 **Makes approx. 10 cups, combined pasta and sauce (4 servings)** 〛
Serving size: Approx. 1 cup pasta with approx. 1⅓ cups sauce

4 qts.	water
1 tbs.	coarse salt
6 oz.	spaghetti (approx. ⅓ box)
1 lb.	tomatoes-on-the-vine, seeds removed and sliced into bite-sized pieces[1]
6 oz.	fresh mozzarella, cut into bite-sized cubes
20	fresh basil leaves, hand-ripped into small pieces
2 tbs.	olive oil
	salt to taste, optional

1. Bring 4 quarts water to a rolling boil in a large pot. Add salt.
2. Add the spaghetti to boiling water. Stir until all strands are completely submerged.
3. Once water returns to a boil, cook pasta, uncovered, for 8 minutes, stirring occasionally. DO NOT OVERCOOK.
4. While the pasta is cooking, prepare the tomatoes, mozzarella, and basil and place each in a separate small bowl.
5. When the pasta is cooked al dente, drain and return to pot. Toss with olive oil. Cool slightly.
6. Divide pasta equally into four bowls.
7. For the uncooked sauce: In each of the individual bowls on top of the pasta, prepare 3 concentric circles starting at the outer rim. In the outermost circle, form a large border of cut tomatoes. Then form a circle of

the cheese cubes. In the center, place a small mound of basil. Sprinkle salt over sauce, if desired. Serve immediately.

GI = LOW   GL = MODERATE
[1] Tomatoes should be ripe but firm.

Just-Plain-Good Pasta

IF you like natural, earthy flavors, this simple recipe is for you.

(**Makes 7 cups   Serving size: 1¾ cups**)

4 qts.	water
1 tbs.	coarse salt
6 oz.	linguine
10 oz.	fresh spinach leaves, stems removed and washed
8 oz.	fresh mushrooms, washed and sliced
1 6-oz. jar	marinated artichoke hearts, drained and thinly sliced
6	whole, peeled, no-salt-added canned tomatoes, cut into thin strips
12	large pitted black olives, halved lengthwise
1 tbs.	olive oil
⅛ tsp.	garlic powder or 2 garlic cloves, freshly minced

1. Bring 4 quarts of water to a rolling boil in a large pot. Add the salt.
2. Add the pasta to boiling water. Stir until all strands are completely submerged.
3. Once water returns to a boil, cook the pasta, uncovered, for 8 minutes, stirring occasionally. DO NOT OVERCOOK.
4. While the pasta is cooking, place the spinach in a strainer and rinse under cold water.
5. Place the spinach in a large skillet with just the water clinging to its leaves. Cover and cook over medium heat for a few minutes until the leaves are wilted. Remove from pan, drain, and set aside.
6. Away from the flame, spray the same pan with vegetable spray, add the mushrooms and sauté for 3 minutes.

7. Return the spinach to the pan and add the artichokes, tomatoes, and olives. Mix well.
8. Drizzle the olive oil over vegetables and stir.
9. When the pasta is cooked, drain well and add to the vegetables in the pan, sprinkle garlic powder or minced garlic. Toss thoroughly. Serve immediately.

EACH SERVING CONTAINS:
303 calories, 51 grams carbohydrate, 10 grams protein, 9 grams fat, 0 milligrams cholesterol, 6 grams fiber

GI = LOW   GL = MODERATE

Red, White, and Green Pan "Pizza"

HAVE you ever seen a cholesterol-free pizza? When you make this recipe, you'll be looking at one! Good for vegetarians, good for kids, good for everyone.

【 Makes 4 servings   Serving Size: ¼ pizza 】

6 oz.	penne pasta
1 tbs.	olive oil
1 clove	garlic, minced
6 cups	shredded zucchini (about 4 medium)
¼ cup	sun-dried tomatoes (about 4 halves)
1 tbs.	extra-virgin olive oil
	cooking spray

1. Cook the pasta according to manufacturer's directions. Remove from heat 1 minute *before* recommended cooking time to keep the pasta al dente (undercooked). Drain the pasta and place it in a large mixing bowl.
2. While the pasta is cooking, heat the oil in a medium skillet and sauté the next 3 ingredients (garlic through sun-dried tomatoes) for 5 minutes over medium-high heat. Stir frequently.
3. Add the vegetables to the pasta in the bowl and toss.
4. Spray a 10″ skillet with cooking spray and heat. Add the extra-virgin olive oil. Pour in the pasta mixture and press down firmly to make it compact. Cook uncovered for 6 minutes on medium heat.
5. Remove from heat. Place a large flat plate over the skillet and flip it over, allowing the "pizza" to loosen onto the plate. Carefully slide it back into the skillet and continue cooking for another 3 minutes, occasionally pressing down firmly on the pasta.
6. When done, use the plate again to remove the "pizza" from the pan.
7. May be served warm or at room temperature.

EACH SERVING CONTAINS:
249 calories, 39 grams carbohydrate, 8 gram protein, 8 grams fat, 0 milligrams cholesterol, 4 grams fiber

GI = LOW   GL = MODERATE

Spaghetti Aglio e Olio Deluxe

THIS is the only pasta recipe I own that does not include vegetables (not that you couldn't add some zucchini and diced tomatoes!) But this recipe allows you to make a wholesome, nutritious dish even when there is "no food in the house."

❨ **Makes 4 cups   Serving size: 1 cup** ❩

2 tbs.	pignoli nuts (½ oz.)
8 oz.	spaghetti
2 tbs.	extra-virgin olive oil
2–3 cloves	garlic, minced
⅓ cup	grated Parmesan cheese
	black pepper, freshly ground, to taste
	red pepper flakes, optional

1. Spread the pignoli nuts in a small skillet. Toast on low heat for 5 minutes, then set aside to cool.
2. Cook the pasta according to package directions.
3. While the pasta is cooking, heat the oil in a small, heavy saucepan, over low heat. Add the garlic and cook approximately 2 to 3 minutes, stirring frequently to prevent burning. Remove the saucepan from the heat.
4. When the pasta is cooked, drain and return it to the pot. Drizzle the oil with garlic over the pasta and mix thoroughly. Add the cheese and the black pepper; mix well.
5. Distribute the pasta into four plates and top with pignoli nuts, and red pepper if you wish. Serve immediately.

EACH SERVING CONTAINS:
319 calories, 42 grams carbohydrate, 11grams protein, 12 grams fat, 6 milligrams cholesterol, 2 grams fiber

GI = LOW   GL = MODERATE

Bowties with Creamed Mushrooms

THE creamy texture and the blend of the earthy flavors from the mushrooms and the brandy make this dish an absolute gourmet pleasure. And nobody would guess that it is low in fat!

{ **Makes 6 servings   Serving size: 1½ cups** }

2 tbs.	tub margarine or butter, separated
10 oz.	fresh mushrooms, cleaned and sliced[1]
¼ cup	brandy or marsala wine
½ cup	vegetable broth, if needed
10 oz.	bowtie pasta
4 wedges	light spreadable cheese[2]
¼ cup	grated Parmesan cheese
½ cup	evaporated skim milk
	nutmeg (optional)

1. Melt 1 tablespoon of margarine (or butter) in a non-stick skillet, add the mushrooms and the brandy (or wine). Cook over high heat for 2 minutes until the alcohol has evaporated. Cover and simmer for 20 minutes, adding vegetable broth if needed.
2. Meanwhile, cook the pasta according to package directions.
3. While the pasta is cooking, mix the remaining margarine and the next 3 ingredients (cheese wedges through evaporated milk) in a wide pan or Dutch oven. Simmer while stirring until a smooth cream forms (about 5 minutes).
4. Drain the cooked pasta. Add to the mushroom mixture. Toss well. Tap with a sprinkle of nutmeg if desired. Serve immediately.

188

> **EACH SERVING CONTAINS:**
> 269 calories, 41 grams carbohydrate, 11 grams protein, 6 grams fat, 8 milligrams cholesterol, 2 grams fiber

GI = LOW   **GL = MODERATE**

[1] Use your favorite kind or even a blend of several kinds (like champignon, morels, shitake, or chanterelles).

[2] Look for brands like Laughing Cow or Swiss Knight in the dairy section of your supermarket.

Luscious Lentil Lasagna

HERE is a power-packed lunch or dinner entrée that may just become a standard in your menu repertoire. Lasagna? Easy to make? This one is!

{ **Makes 8 servings   Serving size: ⅛ pan** }

24 oz.	vegetable broth
½ cup	lentils, washed
½ tbs.	olive or canola oil
2	scallions, coarsely chopped
1 large clove	garlic, minced
1 15-oz. can	diced tomatoes
1 cup	tomato sauce
9 oz.	lasagna noodles, oven ready
16 oz.	lite ricotta
12 oz.	part skim mozzarella, shredded
¼ cup	freshly grated Parmesan cheese
	cooking spray

1. Preheat the oven to 350°.
2. Bring the broth to a boil in a small saucepan. Add the lentils, cover and simmer for 30 minutes, stirring occasionally.
3. While the lentils are cooking, prepare the sauce: place the oil in a heated skillet; add the scallions and the garlic; sauté for 3 minutes or until translucent.
4. When the lentils are cooked, pour them and any remaining liquid into the skillet. Add the tomatoes and the tomato sauce. Stir well. Return the skillet to the heat, cover and simmer for 30 minutes.
5. In the meantime, soften the noodles in a bowl with hot water for about 7 to 8 minutes.
6. In a greased 9″ × 13″ baking pan, prepare the layers as follows:
   - 1 to 2 tablespoons of tomato sauce on the bottom of the pan
   - 4 lasagna noodles, overlapping

- ¹/₂ cup of ricotta
- ¹/₄ of the lentil-tomato sauce
- ³/₄ cup of mozzarella
- 1 tablespoon of grated cheese

7. Repeat for 3 more layers. Cover with foil and bake for 30 to 40 minutes. Remove the pan from the oven and let it rest, covered, for 15 minutes, before serving.

> **EACH SERVING CONTAINS:**
> 405 calories, 41 grams carbohydrate, 26grams protein, 15 grams fat, 76 milligrams cholesterol, 6 grams fiber

GI = LOW   **GL = MODERATE**

Tortellini and Ham Salad

THERE are unlimited variations to this basic recipe to suit anyone's preferred tastes. It can be prepared ahead of time and works well for leftovers, too. The unusually high fat content comes primarily from the heart-healthy olive oil.

(Makes 15 cups   Serving size: 1½ cups)

3 tbs.	extra-virgin olive oil
2 tbs.	red wine vinegar
1 lb.	cheese tortellini, cooked and drained
6 cups	fresh broccoli florets, cooked[1]
3 cups	red bell peppers (2 large), cut into 1" julienne strips[2]
½ cup	red onion, coarsely chopped
2 14-oz. cans	artichoke hearts, drained and quartered
4 oz.	rosemary ham, cut into 2" strips[3]

1. Combine the oil and vinegar in a small jar and shake well. Set aside.
2. Add the remaining ingredients (tortellini through ham) to a large serving bowl. Pour in the dressing and toss well. Serve at room temperature.

EACH SERVING CONTAINS:
208 calories, 23 grams carbohydrate, 8 grams protein, 8 grams fat, 23 milligrams cholesterol, 3grams fiber

GI = LOW   GL = LOW

[1] Use frozen broccoli cuts to save time. Microwave on high for 5 minutes.

[2] Use 1½ cups of roasted peppers from a jar, if preferred.

[3] Substitute low-salt ham, or turkey, or grilled chicken breast if preferred.

Goat Cheese Wrap

HERE'S a quick grab-and-run sandwich. You can prepare it the night before and seal it tightly with plastic wrap. It'll taste great the next day.

❨ Makes 4 wraps   Serving size: 1 wrap ❩

4 oz.	crumbled goat cheese
6	kalamata olives, coarsely chopped
¼ cup	marinated sun-dried tomatoes, thinly sliced
¼ cup	red onion, coarsely chopped
1 tsp.	olive oil
2 tsp.	balsamic vinegar
1 cup	arugula leaves (approx. 20)
8 1-oz. slices	low-salt boiled ham
4 2-oz.	tortillas

1. Combine the first 6 ingredients (goat cheese through vinegar) in medium bowl; set aside.
2. Chop the arugula leaves, set aside.
3. Arrange 2 slices of ham on each tortilla, overlapping them and placing them close to one end.
4. Spoon one-quarter of the cheese mixture on ham.
5. Top each tortilla with ¼ cup arugula leaves.
6. Starting at end with the ham and cheese, completely roll up the tortilla.
7. May be prepared and refrigerated several hours in advance or overnight.

EACH SERVING CONTAINS:
300 calories, 30 grams carbohydrate, 19 grams protein, 11 grams fat, 55 milligrams cholesterol, 2 grams fiber

GI = MODERATE   GL = MODERATE

Vinaigrette Asparagus with Eggs

THIS is a simple, inexpensive, wholesome dish that is as pleasant to look at as it is to taste. A definite crowd-pleaser, this dish is a common main dish in several Mediterranean countries.

〔 **Makes approx. 45 thin spears   Serving size: approx. 15 thin spears** 〕

1 bunch	thin fresh asparagus (approx.12 oz.)
3	hard-boiled eggs, shelled and quartered
	salt and pepper, to taste
	vinaigrette dressing (1 tbs. olive oil, ½ tsp red wine vinegar, salt, and pepper to taste, whisked together)
¼ cup	grated Parmesan cheese

1. Cut or break off 2" from the bottom of the asparagus stalks. Wash and place them in a steam basket with 1" of water in a saucepan. Cover and steam until tender (thin asparagus need about 3 minutes—thick asparagus may require 10 to 12 minutes)
2. In the meantime, in a small bowl lightly mash the eggs with a fork; add salt and pepper to taste. Set aside.
3. Place the cooked asparagus in a deep, oblong serving dish. Toss with the vinaigrette dressing and the grated cheese.
4. Arrange eggs on top of the asparagus. Serve warm.

EACH SERVING CONTAINS:
165 calories, 5 grams carbohydrates, 11 grams protein, 11 grams fat, 215 milligrams cholesterol, 2 grams fiber

GI = LOW   GL = LOW

Snacks

Pizzette ("Little Pizzas")

THIS is a wholesome, satisfying and nourishing snack for kids and grown-ups alike. It takes almost no time to prepare and watch how it disappears in no time, too!

【 Makes 1 serving 】

1	100% whole wheat English muffin, halved
2 tbs.	pizza sauce
2 tbs. (1 oz.)	part skim mozzarella cheese, shredded
Sprinkle	dried oregano

1. Place the muffin halves outside up on a baking sheet. Broil 4½" from heat for 2 minutes.
2. Remove the muffins and turn them over. Spread a tablespoon of pizza sauce on each half and then sprinkle with the cheese and the oregano.
3. Return to oven for approximately 1 minute, or until the cheese has melted. Serve immediately.

EACH SERVING CONTAINS:
210 calories, 24 grams carbohydrate, 13 grams protein, 7 grams fat, 16 milligrams cholesterol, 3 grams fiber

GI = LOW   GL = MODERATE

Cherry-Oat Crunchies

WHO doesn't love cookies? How about cookies that your body will love too? Here they are! Add them to brown-bag lunches, or have with a glass of milk after school or in the evening. Make an extra batch because these cookies will disappear fast!

{ **Makes 42 cookies   Serving size: 2 cookies** }

¼ cup	light brown sugar
¼ cup	honey
½ cup	tub margarine or light butter (4 oz.)
1	egg
¼ cup	egg substitute
½ tsp.	baking soda
½ tbs.	vanilla
1 cup	whole wheat flour
2 cups	rolled oats
1 cup	fresh cherries, pitted and coarsely chopped (approx. 20)[1]
½ cup	walnuts, coarsely chopped
2 cups	bran flakes cereal, crushed
	cooking spray

1. Preheat oven to 350°F.
2. Place the first 7 ingredients (brown sugar through vanilla) in a large mixing bowl. Beat on medium speed for 2 minutes.
3. Fold in the next 5 ingredients (flour through cereal). Mix thoroughly.
4. Spray 2 baking sheets with cooking spray. Drop cookie batter by the tablespoon, about 2" apart.
5. Bake 15 minutes, until lightly brown.
6. Let the cookies cool about 5 minutes, before removing.

EACH SERVING CONTAINS:
132 calories, 18 grams carbohydrate, 3 grams protein, 6 grams fat, 9 milligrams cholesterol, 2 grams fiber

GI = LOW   GL = LOW
[1] You can try other fresh fruit in season or substitute ½ cup of dried fruit.

Chocolate Applesauce Cupcake

YOU just can't imagine how light and moist and good-tasting these cupcakes are unless you try them. Any nutritionist would agree that eating one of these treats is 179 calories well "spent."

❰ **Makes 12 large or 48 mini cupcakes**

Serving size: 1 large cupcake or 4 mini cupcakes ❱

½ cup	tub margarine or light butter
¾ cup	sugar
1	egg
¼ cup	egg substitute
½ cup	cocoa powder, unsweetened
1½ cup	natural applesauce
1¾ cup	whole wheat flour
1 tsp.	baking powder
1 tsp.	baking soda
½ tsp.	salt

1. Preheat oven to 350°F. Grease and flour a 12-cupcake tin.
2. In a deep mixing bowl, cream the margarine (or butter) and the sugar (about $1^{1}/_{2}$ minutes at medium speed).
3. Add in the egg, egg substitute, and cocoa powder, and mix until smooth (approximately 1 minute, scraping sides frequently). Fold in the applesauce.
4. In a small mixing bowl, combine the next 4 ingredients (flour through salt). Add the dry ingredients to the egg mixture and combine by hand, using about 60 to 70 strokes. Do not over mix.
5. Fill the cupcake molds half to three-quarters full. Bake the large cupcakes for 22 minutes and the mini cupcakes for 15 minutes. Cool before removing from pan.

EACH SERVING CONTAINS:
186 calories, 31 grams carbohydrate, 4 grams protein; 7 grams fat, 18 milligrams cholesterol, 4 grams fiber

GI = LOW   **GL = MODERATE**

Chocolate-Pear Smoothie

THIRTY seconds to prepare, thirty seconds to mix, and then take your time to enjoy this luscious, creamy treat.

❨ **Makes 2 servings   Serving size: 12 oz.** ❩

8 oz.	nonfat or 1% milk
2 tbs.	unsweetened cocoa powder
1	pear (fresh, frozen or canned) peeled and cut into small pieces
1 tsp.	honey
Dash	ground cardamom (optional)

1. Combine all ingredients in a food processor. Blend at high speed for 30 seconds.

2. Pour into two 12-oz. glasses. Serve immediately.

EACH SERVING CONTAINS:
131 calories, 27 grams carbohydrate, 6 grams protein, 2 grams fat; 0 milligrams cholesterol, 3 grams fiber

GI = LOW   GL = LOW

Simply Delicious Applesauce

HERE'S a perfect example in cooking when less is *definitely* more. The only simpler way to eat an apple is straight off the tree!

〖 **Makes 5 ½ cups   Serving size: ½ cup** 〗

4 lbs.	mixed apples (Gala, Macintosh, Rome Beauty, Cortland)
1 tbs.	vanilla extract
1 tsp.	cinnamon

1. Core and peel the apples. Slice them into eighths and then cut them in half horizontally.
2. Place the apple chunks into a wide-based pot and cover. Do not add water.
3. Cook over medium-low heat for approximately 30 minutes or until the mixture reaches desired consistency. Stir every few minutes to prevent sticking.
4. Remove the apples from heat.
5. Add in the vanilla and cinnamon and mix thoroughly.
6. May be served warm or cold.
7. Store in refrigerator.

EACH SERVING CONTAINS:
95 calories, 23 grams carbohydrate, less than 1 gram protein, less than 1 gram fat, 0 milligrams cholesterol, 3 grams fiber

GI = LOW   GL = LOW

Appendix:
The Glycemic Index Values
of Some Popular Foods

As you look over the list on the following pages, keep in mind that I classify a food's glycemic index value this way:

Trickler carbs	low GI (0–55)*
Moderate carbs	(56–69)
Gusher carbs	high GI (70 or greater)

* Numbers refer to glycemic index scale based on 0–100.

FOOD	LOW	MODERATE	HIGH

BAKERY PRODUCTS

Cakes

FOOD	LOW	MODERATE	HIGH
Banana	○		
Chocolate, with chocolate frosting	○		
Pound	○		
Sponge	○		
Vanilla	○		
Angel food		◑	
Flan		◑	

Muffins

FOOD	LOW	MODERATE	HIGH
Apple with sugar or artificial sweeteners	○		
Apple, oat, and raisin	○		
Banana, oat and honey		◑	
Bran		◑	
Blueberry		◑	
Carrot		◑	
Oatmeal, made from mix, Quaker Oats		◑	
Cupcake, iced			●
Scone, plain			●

Pastries

FOOD	LOW	MODERATE	HIGH
Croissant		◑	
Doughnut, cake-type			●

BEVERAGES

Alcoholic

FOOD	LOW	MODERATE	HIGH
Beer	○		
Brandy	○		
Gin	○		
Sherry	○		
Whiskey	○		
Wine, red	○		
Wine, white	○		

FOOD	LOW	MODERATE	HIGH
Juices			
Apple, with sugar or artificial sweetener	○		
Carrot, fresh	○		
Grapefruit, unsweetened	○		
Pineapple, unsweetened	○		
Tomato, canned, no added sugar	○		
Smoothies and Shakes			
Raspberry	○		
Soy	○		
Soft Drinks			
Coke		◑	
Fanta®		◑	
Sports drinks			
Gatorade®			●

BREADS

FOOD	LOW	MODERATE	HIGH
Fruit			
Muesli, made from mix	○		
Happiness™, cinnamon, raisin, pecan		◑	
Gluten-free			
Fiber-enriched			●
White			●
Rye			
Pumpernickel	○		
Sourdough	○		
Cocktail		◑	
Light		◑	
Whole wheat		◑	
Spelt			
Multigrain	○		
White			●

FOOD	LOW	MODERATE	HIGH
Wheat			
100% stone-ground whole wheat	○		
100% whole grain	○		
Soy & linseed bread machine mix	○		
Flatbread, Indian		◑	
Hearty 7-grain		◑	
Pita, plain		◑	
Bagel			●
Baguette			●
Bread stuffing			●
English muffin			●
Flatbread, Middle Eastern			●
Italian			●
Lebanese, white			●
White, enriched			●
Whole wheat			●

BREAKFAST FOODS

FOOD	LOW	MODERATE	HIGH
Breakfast cereal bars			
Rice Krispies Treat		◑	
Cooked cereals			
Hot cereal, apple & cinnamon, Con Agra	○		
Old-fashioned oats	○		
Cream of Wheat™, regular, Nabisco		◑	
One Minute Oats, Quaker Oats		◑	
Quick Oats, Quaker Oats		◑	
Cream of Wheat™, instant, Nabisco			●
Oatmeal, instant			●
Grain products			
Pancakes, prepared from mix	○		
Pancakes, buckwheat, gluten-free, made from mix			●
Waffles, Aunt Jemima®			●

FOOD	LOW	MODERATE	HIGH
Ready-to-eat cereals			
All-Bran®, Kellogg's	○		
Complete™ Bran Flakes, Kellogg's	○		
Bran Buds™, Kellogg's		◐	
Bran Chex™, Kellogg's		◐	
Froot Loops™, Kellogg's		◐	
Frosted Flakes™, Kellogg's		◐	
Just Right™, Kellogg's		◐	
Life™, Quaker Oats		◐	
Nutrigrain™, Kellogg's		◐	
Oat bran, raw, Quaker Oats		◐	
Puffed Wheat, Quaker Oats		◐	
Raisin Bran™, Kellogg's		◐	
Special K™, Kellogg's		◐	
Bran Flakes™, Kellogg's			●
Cheerios™, General Mills			●
Corn Chex™, Kellogg's			●
Corn Flakes™, Kellogg's			●
Corn Pops™, Kellogg's			●
Grapenuts™, Post			●
Rice Krispies™, Kellogg's			●
Shredded Wheat™, Nabisco			●
Team™ Flakes, Nabisco			●
Total™			●
Weetabix™			●

COOKIES

FOOD	LOW	MODERATE	HIGH
Hearty Oatmeal, Fifty 50	○		
Oatmeal, Sugar-Free, Fifty 50	○		
Social Tea Biscuits	○		
Vanilla wafers, creme filled, Fifty 50	○		
Arrowroot		◐	
Digestives		◐	
Shortbread		◐	
Vanilla wafers			●

FOOD	LOW	MODERATE	HIGH

CRACKERS

FOOD	LOW	MODERATE	HIGH
Breton wheat		◑	
Melba Toast		◑	
Rye crispbread		◑	
Ryvita™		◑	
Stoned Wheat Thins		◑	
Water		◑	
Kavli™ Norwegian Crispbread			●
Premium soda (Saltines)			●
Rice cakes, puffed			●

DAIRY PRODUCTS AND ALTERNATIVES

Custard
FOOD	LOW	MODERATE	HIGH
Homemade	○		

Ice cream
FOOD	LOW	MODERATE	HIGH
Regular	○		

Milk
FOOD	LOW	MODERATE	HIGH
Low-fat, chocolate, with aspartame	○		
Low-fat, chocolate, with sugar	○		
Skim	○		
Whole	○		
Condensed, sweetened			●

Mousse
FOOD	LOW	MODERATE	HIGH
Butterscotch, low-fat, Nestlé	○		
Chocolate, low-fat, Nestlé	○		
French vanilla, low-fat, Nestlé	○		
Hazelnut, low-fat, Nestlé	○		
Mango, low-fat, Nestlé	○		
Mixed berry, low-fat, Nestlé	○		
Strawberry, low-fat, Nestlé	○		

Pudding
FOOD	LOW	MODERATE	HIGH
Instant, chocolate, made with milk	○		
Instant, vanilla, made with milk	○		

FOOD	LOW	MODERATE	HIGH
Soy milk			
Reduced fat	○		
Whole	○		
Soy yogurt			
Tofu-based frozen dessert, chocolate			●
Yogurt			
Low-fat, fruit, with aspartame	○		
Low-fat, fruit, with sugar	○		
Nonfat, French vanilla, with sugar	○		
Nonfat, strawberry, with sugar	○		

FRUIT AND FRUIT PRODUCTS

FOOD	LOW	MODERATE	HIGH
Apple, fresh	○		
Apricot, fresh	○		
Banana, fresh	○		
Cantaloupe, fresh	○		
Cherries, fresh	○		
Grapefruit, fresh	○		
Grapes, fresh	○		
Kiwi, fresh	○		
Mango, fresh	○		
Orange, fresh	○		
Peach, canned in natural juice	○		
Peach, fresh	○		
Pear, canned in pear juice	○		
Pear, fresh	○		
Plum, fresh	○		
Prunes, pitted	○		
Strawberries, fresh	○		
Strawberry jam	○		
Figs, dried		◑	
Fruit cocktail, canned		◑	
Papaya, fresh		◑	
Peach, canned in heavy syrup		◑	
Peach, canned in light syrup		◑	
Pineapple, fresh		◑	
Raisins/sultanas		◑	

FOOD	LOW	MODERATE	HIGH
Dates, dried			●
Lychee, canned in syrup, drained			●
Watermelon, fresh			●

GRAINS

FOOD	LOW	MODERATE	HIGH
Barley, cracked	○		
Barley, pearled	○		
Buckwheat	○		
Buckwheat groats	○		
Bulgur	○		
Corn, canned, no salt added	○		
Rice, brown	○		
Rice, Cajun Style, Uncle Ben's®	○		
Rice, Long Grain and Wild, Uncle Ben's®	○		
Rice, parboiled, converted, white, cooked 20–30 min, Uncle Ben's®	○		
Barley, rolled		◐	
Corn, fresh		◐	
Cornmeal		◐	
Couscous		◐	
Rice, arborio (risotto)		◐	
Rice, basmati		◐	
Rice, Garden Style, Uncle Ben's®		◐	
Rice, parboiled, long grain, cooked 10 minutes		◐	
Millet			●
Rice, sticky			●
Rice, parboiled			●
Tapioca boiled with milk			●

INFANT FORMULA AND BABY FOODS

Baby foods

FOOD	LOW	MODERATE	HIGH
Apple, apricot, and banana, baby cereal		◐	
Chicken and noodles with vegetables, strained		◐	
Corn and rice, baby		◐	
Oatmeal, creamed, baby		◐	
Rice pudding, baby		◐	

FOOD	LOW	MODERATE	HIGH

Infant formula

SMA, 20 cal./fl oz, Wyeth	○		
Nursoy, soy-based, milk-free, Wyeth		◑	

LEGUMES

Beans

Baked, canned	○		
Butter, dried and cooked	○		
Kidney, canned	○		
Lima, baby, frozen	○		
Mung, cooked	○		
Navy, dried and cooked	○		
Pinto, cooked	○		
Soy, canned	○		

Lentils

Green, dried and cooked	○		
Red, dried and cooked	○		

Peas

Black-eyed	○		
Chickpeas/garbanzo beans, canned	○		
Split, yellow, cooked	○		

MEAL-REPLACEMENT PRODUCTS

Designer chocolate, sugar-free, Worldwide Sport Nutrition low-carbohydrate products	○		
L.E.A.N Fibergy™ bar, Harvest Oat, Usana	○		
L.E.A.N (Life long) Nutribar™, Peanut Crunch, Usana	○		
L.E.A.N (Life long) Nutribar™, Chocolate Crunch, Usana	○		

MIXED MEALS AND CONVENIENCE FOODS

Chicken nuggets, frozen, reheated	○		
Fish fillet, reduced fat, breaded	○		

FOOD	LOW	MODERATE	HIGH
Fish sticks	○		
Greek lentil stew with a bread roll, homemade	○		
Lean Cuisine™, chicken with rice	○		
Pizza, Super Supreme, pan, Pizza Hut	○		
Pizza, Super Supreme, thin and crispy, Pizza Hut	○		
Pizza, Vegetarian Supreme, thin and crispy, Pizza Hut	○		
Spaghetti Bolognese	○		
Sushi, salmon	○		
Tortellini, cheese, Stouffer	○		
Tuna patty, reduced fat	○		
Cheese sandwich, white bread		◑	
Kugel		◑	
Macaroni and cheese, boxed, Kraft		◑	
Peanut-butter sandwich, white/whole wheat bread		◑	
Pizza, cheese, Pillsbury		◑	
Spaghetti, gluten-free, canned in tomato sauce		◑	
Sushi, roasted sea algae, vinegar, and rice		◑	
Taco shells, cornmeal-based, baked, El Paso		◑	
White bread and butter		◑	
Stir-fried vegetables with chicken and rice, homemade			●

NOODLES

FOOD	LOW	MODERATE	HIGH
Instant	○		
Mung bean, Lungkow beanthread	○		
Rice, fresh, cooked	○		
Rice, dried, cooked		◑	
Udon, plain, reheated 5 min.		◑	

PASTA

FOOD	LOW	MODERATE	HIGH
Capellini	○		
Fettuccine, egg	○		
Gluten-free, cornstarch	○		
Linguine, thick, fresh, durum wheat, white	○		
Linguine, thin, fresh, durum wheat	○		

FOOD	LOW	MODERATE	HIGH
Macaroni, plain, cooked	○		
Ravioli	○		
Spaghetti, cooked 5 min.	○		
Spaghetti, cooked 22 min.	○		
Spaghetti, protein enriched, cooked 7 min.	○		
Spaghetti, whole wheat	○		
Spirali, cooked, durum wheat	○		
Star pastina, cooked 5 min.	○		
Tortellini	○		
Vermicelli	○		
Gnocchi		◑	
Rice vermicelli		◑	
Spaghetti, cooked 10 min., Barilla		◑	
Corn, gluten-free			●
Rice and corn, gluten-free			●
Rice, brown, cooked 16 min.			●

PROTEIN FOODS

FOOD	LOW	MODERATE	HIGH
Beef	○		
Cheese	○		
Cold cuts	○		
Eggs	○		
Fish	○		
Lamb	○		
Pork	○		
Sausages	○		
Shellfish (shrimp, crab, lobster, etc.)	○		
Veal	○		

SNACK FOODS AND CANDY

Candy

FOOD	LOW	MODERATE	HIGH
Nougat	○		
Jelly beans			●
Life Savers®			●
Skittles®			●

FOOD	LOW	MODERATE	HIGH
Chips			
Corn, plain, salted, Doritos™	○		
Potato, plain, salted	○		
Chocolate bars			
Milk, Cadbury's	○		
Milk, Dove®, Mars	○		
Milk, Nestlé	○		
White, Milky Bar®	○		
Mars Bar®		◑	
Snickers Bar®		◑	
Chocolate candy			
M & M's®, peanut	○		
Chocolate spread			
Nutella®, chocolate hazelnut spread	○		
Dried fruit bars			
Fruit Roll-Ups®			●
Nuts			
Cashews	○		
Peanuts	○		
Pecans	○		
Popcorn			
Plain, microwaved			●
Pretzels			
Plain, salted			●
Snack bars			
Apple Cinnamon, Con Agra	○		
Peanut Butter & Choc-Chip	○		
Twix® Cookie Bar, caramel	○		
Kudos Whole Grain Bars, chocolate chip		◑	

FOOD	LOW	MODERATE	HIGH
Sports bars			
Ironman PR bar®, chocolate	○		
PowerBar®, chocolate		◑	

SOUPS

Lentil, canned	○		
Minestrone, canned, ready-to-serve	○		
Tomato, canned	○		
Black bean, canned		◑	
Green pea, canned		◑	
Split pea, canned		◑	

SPECIAL DIETARY PRODUCTS

Choice DM™, vanilla, Mead Johnson	○		
Ensure™, Abbott	○		
Ensure Plus™, vanilla, Abbott	○		
Ensure Pudding™, vanilla, Abbott	○		
Ensure™ bar, chocolate fudge brownie, Abbott	○		
Ensure™, vanilla, Abbott	○		
Glucerna™ bar, lemon crunch, Abbott	○		
Glucerna™ SR shake, vanilla, Abbott	○		
Glucerna™, vanilla, Abbott	○		
Resource Diabetic™, vanilla, Novartis	○		
Resource Plus, chocolate, Novartis	○		
Ultracal™ with fiber, Mead Johnson	○		
Enercal Plus™, Wyeth-Ayerst		◑	
Enrich Plus shake, vanilla, Ross		◑	

SUGARS

Blue Agave, Organic Agave Cactus Nectar, light, 90% fructose, Western Commerce	○		
Blue Agave, Organic Agave Cactus Nectar, light, 97% fructose, Western Commerce	○		
Fructose	○		
Lactose	○		

FOOD	LOW	MODERATE	HIGH
Honey		◑	
Sucrose		◑	
Glucose			●
Maltose			●

VEGETABLES

FOOD	LOW	MODERATE	HIGH
Artichokes	○		
Avocado	○		
Bok choy	○		
Broccoli	○		
Cabbage	○		
Carrots, peeled, cooked	○		
Cassava (yuca), cooked with salt	○		
Cauliflower	○		
Celery	○		
Corn, canned, no salt added	○		
Cucumber	○		
French beans (runner beans)	○		
Leafy greens	○		
Lettuce	○		
Peas, frozen, cooked	○		
Pepper	○		
Potato, sweet	○		
Squash	○		
Yam	○		
Beet		◑	
Corn, sweet, cooked		◑	
Potato, boiled/canned		◑	
Potato, new, canned		◑	
Taro		◑	
Broad beans			●
Parsnips			●
Potato, French fries, frozen and reheated			●
Potato, instant			●
Potato, mashed			●

FOOD	LOW	MODERATE	HIGH
Potato, microwaved			●
Potato, russet, baked			●
Pumpkin			●
Rutabaga			●

GI list reprinted and adapted from *The New Glucose Revolution Complete Guide to Glycemic Index Values,* courtesy of Marlowe & Company.

ACKNOWLEDGMENTS

Hide not your talents, they for use were made.
What's a sun-dial in the shade?
—Benjamin Franklin

- Linda Rao, for her insightful contributions to the first edition of *Good Carbs, Bad Carbs*.
- Peter Jacoby, Pauline Neuwirth, and the editorial and design staffs of the Avalon Publishing Group for helping me keep the bar raised through their skills, intelligence, patience, and understanding.
- Marie Brown, Laura Garrett, M.S., R.D., C.D.E., Barbara Halma, R.N., Richard Berkowitz, M.D., and Kenneth Lubansky, M.D., for generously sharing their thoughts and expertise with me.
- Maria Gill for decades of cooking and sharing recipes with me.
- Lucy and Camille for their unconditional love.
- Matthew Lore, for his belief in the glycemic index message and in my ability to contribute to it.
- The pioneer scientists in Canada and Australia for creating and expanding the Glycemic Index, which has helped so many people lead healthier lives.
- My wonderful patients, who generously share their courage and wisdom with me every day.

INDEX

About the Author

JOHANNA BURANI, M.S., R.D., C.D.E., is a Registered Dietitian and Certified Diabetes Educator with nearly two decades of
experience in nutritional counseling. The author of several books
and professional manuals, including *The New Glucose Revolution
Life Plan* (with Dr. Jennie Brand-Miller and Kaye Foster-Powell)
and several pocket guides from the New Glucose Revolution
series, she specializes in patient-empowerment strategies based on
low-GI food choices. She lives in Mendham, New Jersey.